Piece by Piece

Love in the Land of Alzheimer's

by

Susan Tereba

© 2016

Published by

World on a String

Cover Design by Susan Tereba

ISBN - 9780692765678

To Bob

What a dream life we lived!

And to the millions of caregivers of people suffering from dementia

Man becomes mature the moment he starts loving rather than needing.
He starts overflowing, sharing: he starts giving
And when two mature persons are in love, one of the greatest paradoxes of life happens, One of the most beautiful phenomena:
They are together and yet tremendously alone
They are together so much so that they are almost one

-Osho

Table of Contents

Prologue

I started writing this as an article on grieving the loss of Bob, my soulmate and husband, to Alzheimer's, hoping it would bring solace to other caregivers in despair of losing a loved one to this terrible disease. I'd found that by reading other people's experiences on this journey, I didn't feel so alone or guilty for my anger, shortcomings, and especially my impatience.

I didn't realize at the time that this article would become a book, but it kept writing itself. Five years later it was finished. It helped me remember who the man I married was, while I experienced who he'd become. Being his primary caregiver for ten years and then overseeing his care for another four blinded me to his essence. Writing and remembering brought him back to me.

In the year 2000 I had a life-threatening medical emergency. On the fourth day of searing pain it was diagnosed as a stranlated intestine. Bob was convinced that all I needed was a laxative. My knight in shining armor, my protector, my support, my best friend, my lover and business partner was paralyzed, unable to make the simplest decisions, unable even to dial the phone as I teetered on the brink of death.

It was then that our friends knew something was terribly wrong. Bob's reaction to this crisis signaled the initial signs of dementia that would take us first through a speculation that he had Mild Cognitive Impairment, then the dreaded diagnosis five years later that he had Alzheimer's disease.

I faced this diagnosis with a commitment to make Bob's life as good as it could be under the circumstances and to keep him home with me as long as possible. I educated myself about Alzheimer's by reading, Googling, and asking questions. Friends sent me the latest studies. I found a doctor I could trust. I read books about how to be a good caregiver. But I often felt like I was reinventing the wheel.

I futilely fought for Bob with large doses of supplements geared for the brain, mental and physical exercises, and an even healthier diet than we were already eating. I hoped he could avoid the same outcome as his mother and two aunts, who spent their last years in a nursing home tied to chairs, completely demented. Bob's only sibling, a sister three years older, also died of the disease. He'd lived with this fear gnawing at the back of his mind for decades. Then it became his reality.

This is the story of dreams lived, of inner and outer travels, and above all, love. I've changed some of the character's names to protect their privacy but the events are still as I remember them.

Chapter One
Coming to Terms

Let me not pray to be sheltered from dangers,
But to be fearless in facing them
Let me not beg for the stilling of my pain,
But for the heart to conquer it
Let me not crave in anxious fear to be saved
But hope for the patience to win my freedom.

- Rabindranath Tagore

The elegant curves of Chiesa Santo Spirito dominate the Piazza. Magnetically, they beckon me across the threshold of this Renaissance church. Its high arches cascade towards the altar, drawing me deeper into the interior to absorb the beauty of the artistic masterpieces within. I walk quietly, not wanting to disturb the stillness imbued in these timeworn walls.

I find an empty pew and drink in the hush of this sacred space – a space filled with curls of frankincense, whispers of rosaries, and centuries of devotion. Without warning, tears sting my eyes and roll down my cheeks, pooling on my chin.

There's no sobbing, only silent tears of grief held in check for years while I've kept everything together, deflecting whatever challenges have come charging my way. This grief hijacks my precious, laboriously-earned time of joy and respite.

Pain radiates out from my core, filling every cell in my body. It grabs my attention and holds me in its grip, not allowing anything else to enter. Emotionally flailing, I can't seem to catch my breath, or to see the light.

I struggle to right myself with reminders of all I have to be grateful for: that I'm here in Florence, Italy, living a long held dream; that I've been well loved; that my soulmate and I found each other twenty-six years ago. These reminders are in vain. Their ropes of safety slip through my fingers. There is only this pain and these tears.

I sit for what feels like eternity.

Finally, sweet surrender takes me by the hand and I relax into it, allowing the release to take its course. I surf the wave that radiates out from the center of my chest, feeling the feelings without analysis, and sensing that this experience is as sacred as the place I'm in. It becomes a meditation, and a prayer for the courage to face this pain and not shy away from it.

This meditation carries my heart homeward to Bali, the 'Island of the Gods', one of over 17,000 islands in the vast Indonesian archipelago. Indonesia, the fourth largest country in the world, is ninety percent Muslim while the small island of Bali is ninety percent Hindu. The entire archipelago, regardless of religious affiliation, is at its core animistic, meaning the spirit in everything is worshipped, and most importantly, the spirit of the ancestors. Buddhism, Hinduism, Islam, Taoism and

Christianity are overlaid and incorporated into these ancient, animistic beliefs.

In Hindu Bali, daily offerings are made to these spirits in each family compound to keep the environment harmonious. These offerings might be as simple as squares of fresh banana leaf with mounds of cooked rice, or more complex woven palm leaf trays with flowers and shaved green *pandana* leaf over the ever-present rice. On special days, elaborate offerings are constructed; these might include a tower of fruit embellished with a splayed, crisply roasted duck or chicken, sweet rice flour cakes in iridescent colors, and deep-fried pastries.

I couldn't ask for a better place to live with Alzheimer's. The Balinese are caring, compassionate, and above all, patient. There are few homes or institutions for the elderly outside the family compound in Bali so everyone has the experience of accepting and caring for people with *otak tua*, old brain. Few families would dream of sending the elderly and infirm away.

With seeming interest, our staff listen to Bob's same stories recited day after day. His carers have become masters at tossing out juicy morsels to prod him into revealing the story of his youth, where he resides most of the time. They understand when he demands his shoes, his broom, his scoop, or his flashlight, knowing it's the disease demanding and not the man. Without their help, it would be impossible to keep Bob with me and run our business at the same time.

My desire to give Bob the best quality of life he can have is daily challenged by the reality of living with Alzheimer's. I often feel I have ten balls in the air and am juggling as fast as I can while more balls keep coming at me with lightning speed. I lose patience, snap at Bob, and then feel like a failure, knowing he can't help being who he is and that he has neither the power nor the logic to change his actions and reactions. I wake some mornings with aching teeth from clenching them in the night. My heart beats irregularly and sleep dangles beyond my grasp as challenges and tensions elevate.

I desperately need 'alone time' to refill my tank of creativity, which is running merely on fumes. This creativity is my life's blood, my *raison d'être*. It also powers our livelihood.

As an artist, writer, and jewelry designer, the rigors of running a business, managing thirty employees, and writing a food column for the local expat paper while also being the primary caregiver for Bob have taken their toll. At times I feel I'm barely hanging onto my sanity.

***

The idea for this respite trip to Italy solidified into months of planning and organizing. I sometimes questioned whether all the preparation was worth it. Would I be better off just staying at home? The answer was always the same: "Go!"

The first order of business was to develop a full-time care system for Bob so he could remain at home, where he's happiest. It's where he thrives, with established routines and the familiar faces of those who watch over him. People with Alzheimer's disease need the security that comes with a familiar, patterned life. As simple problem solving becomes an enormous challenge, they need the safety net of trusted caregivers.

I felt as if I was putting a life-sized jigsaw puzzle together, trying to think of everything that needed to be in place, every 'what if?' answered. I had lists, and lists of lists, that seemed to surreptitiously replenish themselves as I crossed items off. I woke in the night with list additions that held sleep hostage until I wrote them down. Then, half an hour later, another would come, and then another, until I had a night of list additions and sleep subtractions with dawn coming hours ahead of schedule. I became so addicted to these lists that if I accomplished something not already written on one, I wrote it down and then crossed it off just so I had a sense that I wasn't pedaling backwards.

Friends were enlisted in case an emergency arose while I was away, friends that could be trusted to keep me abreast of any problems and not try to shepherd me away from aggravating situations. I planned Bob's meals, organized medications, and prepared lists of contacts for everyone involved. The list making mushroomed into lists for the backup team and our staff as well.

Right from our heady, romantic beginning, discovery and travel were a large part of the life Bob and I have shared. Now they're no longer viable or enjoyable for Bob since he's lost the ability to keep track of time and place. He often thinks he's in a different country or thinks it's time for breakfast when it's dinnertime. He can't keep track of currencies and misplaces his money and identification daily.

Sometimes he thinks I'm someone else, like the night we were snuggled in bed, drifting off to sleep, and he suddenly got up. "Where are you going?" I inquired as nonchalantly as possible.

"I have to go home to my wife."

"I am your wife."

"Oh", he said, clumsily slipping back under the covers.

In spite of these disabilities, Bob is happy most of the time.

Sweeping and cleaning our verdant tropical garden has been his passion for the last three years. The trees always comply, dropping copious amounts of leaves throughout the day. Sometimes he comes in while I'm on the computer, carrying a great handful of yellowed leaves just plucked from the lawn, and asks triumphantly, "Guess how many I picked up this morning?"

"Forty-two." I grab a number out of the air.

"Nope. Fifty-four!" He grins, having won the game.

By the time he's done with one end of the garden, the other is strewn once again with paper-thin peach bougainvillea blossoms, ridged yellow starfruit, and other tropical detritus. He has numerous brooms, buckets, and scoops, but they're never enough since he misplaces them throughout the day. "Where's my broom!" he bellows to anyone in earshot. I keep hoping if he has sufficient stock of these items, there'll always be one in sight. He's a master at misplacement.

Our koi pond needs skimming twice daily before feeding the 'whales', as we call them, so big and fat have this rainbow of carp become. Sometimes Bob gets in the pond to gather up the saturated leaves and blossoms that have settled to the floor. He carries on conversations with the multicolored beauties swimming around his legs as he plucks and preens the foliage off the bottom and out of the purple spikes of the water hyacinth plants.

And then there's weeding. My sweet husband sits on the ground cross-legged like a meditating monk, lost to time, carefully pulling out the smallest invader. He does this all on his own, without supervision, spending hours in quiet contemplation and having the occasional hushed conversation with the butterflies and dragonflies that brush past. If we go out during the day, he can't return to the house to change his clothes without stooping to pick up leaves or pluck a miscreant weed. His clothes read like a road map with garden stains marking his daily wanderings.

Working with the plants, he's secure in his own world, happy and self-contained. It gives him a sense of accomplishment, purpose, stability, and self-esteem while grounding him tether-like to mother earth. He's at peace in the greenery and he's safe.

But when it rains and he can only venture as far as the veranda, anxiety takes over and he moves inside to organize drawers or shelves again and again. The contents are in constant disarray, which he can never quite come to terms with, and so he often gives up, stuffing everything back into the same or another space, expletives exploding all around him. It must be frightening and frustrating to never be able to rely on things being where he thinks they should be. He concludes someone is stealing from us.

Packing is another compulsive activity and a sure sign of anxiety. I often wake in the morning to find neat piles of bathroom articles stacked for a journey on his chest of drawers or next to the sink. I've even found them tightly bound in a rolled beach towel secured with a rubber band hidden amongst his clothing - a treasury of things that have recently gone missing.

When he can't sleep, he packs. It must comfort him and give him a sense that he'll be prepared for any looming departures, even though he can't remember just where or when the departure will occur. He usually thinks he's going home, and I wonder where that is for him. It saddens me that my husband no longer thinks of our place together as home.

***

"Susan, the band saw!" my assistant, Suarni, called from the jewelry studio in a panicked voice a week or so before I left. I was glued to a project on the computer and it took me a few seconds to float up to the surface. Then it dawned on me what she'd said.

I sprinted out to the workshop. My heart sank. There was Bob cutting a client's piece of expensive fossilized mammoth tusk in half on dangerous equipment. The employees who usually worked there were both out.

Since then, we've had to implement a new rule – the workshop must be locked at all times when the staff are out. This is an inconvenience, to be sure, since the four of us in the office are in and out of there all day long, but it's necessary to keep Bob safe and guard our clients' materials.

This change has distressed Bob. "Susan, I can't open the door!" he bellows, shoving his keys in and out of the lock. While he has two sets of keys, with the hope that he'll always be able to find one of them, they're keys in name only. We've had to surreptitiously take a rasp to them so they won't lock or unlock anything after he locked staff members out of the office a few times.

"There's something wrong with the lock, Bob," I tell him when he tries his keys. "The locksmith is scheduled to come tomorrow." He accepts this and calms down; we have a problem and we're dealing with it. Fortunately, tomorrow never comes for Bob.

Another of the many balls I was juggling before leaving for Italy was the realization that I have to make other sleeping arrangements. After twenty-five years of sleeping together, often holding hands or touching foot to foot, Bob has begun waking me in the dead of night, sitting bold upright, and asking, "Where are we?" or "Now, which way is it to the bathroom?" If I don't wake in time to direct him, he might pee in the kitchen or on a closet door. He's also begun talking clearly and loudly in his sleep, carrying on dialogues with dream companions and leaving me feeling I'm listening in on private conversations. He occasionally strikes out with his hand or fist, hitting me so hard I'm shaken for hours, wide-awake and ready to defend myself. Sharing a bedroom means I'm constantly sleep deprived.

Our small house, which is also our office and studio, has no extra space. It's time to build a separate room for me and train Bob's carers, Ketut and Nano, to take care of his nighttime needs. I'll miss our bedroom and the delicious sensation of settling into the memory foam mattress after a long day. I'll miss Bob's gentle snoring and knowing he's next to me if there's a bump in the night. I'll miss my favorite books being always on hand on the shelf in our headboard and the ritual read before falling asleep.

Changes, hard enough for healthy people, are always a challenge for a person with Alzheimer's. This new arrangement will be difficult for my husband. I know he'll feel abandoned. I know he'll search for me in the night.

One of the survival techniques I've learned as a caregiver is to be as flexible and adaptable as possible while trying to keep my sense of humor. There's a constant letting go of the way our life has been and the way I'd once expected it to continue. I've let go of having my own bath towel, keeping things in their place, and telling the truth. Now it's time to let go of sleeping together in our comfortable bed. A month before I leave for Italy, construction begins on a knockdown coconut wood cabin that will become my new bedroom. Another loss to mourn.

***

This Italian respite trip becomes a carrot tantalizing me to plod – or sometimes gallop - through the mud of the self-elongating lists. I imagine traveling on my own for the first time in twenty-six years, able to move through my days without having to keep constant vigil on Bob's needs and whereabouts or be always attuned to problems that might arise. I imagine what it would be like to get up early to take photographs whenever the mood strikes me, stand with awe in the presence of an Italian masterpiece as long as I desire, or sketch at an outdoor Venetian cafe on the side of a canal. I want to practice my Italian again and immerse myself in the Renaissance. I tell myself I'll go where the wind blows me, making few specific plans. Grief isn't on my agenda, so it comes as a shuddering, time-standing-still shock when it ensnares me time and again throughout the journey with an intensity that could never happen at home.

Death plunges us into a grief that lasts until we come to terms with its finality. Then healing begins and we can move on. The grief that comes with losing someone we love one piece at a time is a protracted loss that engulfs the spirit. Bob is still present physically, a constant reminder of who he once was. My body responds involuntarily to his smells, whether they are after-shower sweet or sweat-induced sharp, to his hand on my arm when he wants my attention, or to verbal expressions so familiar I often use them myself. Sometimes he looks so handsome, his gray-blue eyes dancing as he speaks, that my heart melts and my body has those old, sweet responses even though I know he can never be the husband he was. Subconsciously, the losses have accumulated. In Italy, they become conscious. I feel that the joy of life and my precious alone time are being kidnapped over and over again. The ransom I pay is trying to stay present with the pain, allowing it to be without analyzing it, pushing it away, or hating it. The sooner I embrace and acknowledge it, the sooner the joy returns. The heat of the pain increases the more I resist.

Denial, a much-maligned state of mind, has become a protector on this journey, and I've gained a great respect for it. Where I once scoffed at others in denial of the challenges in their lives, I now see how it's given me breathing space and allowed me to function in difficult situations. It's given me time to gather strength to face what is really happening in each phase of Alzheimer's. I need all that strength to endure the pain, and hopefully endure it with grace.

I've observed a pattern emerging. Each time Bob reaches a plateau and his symptoms stabilize, I adapt to them and accept them almost as normal. Then he begins bumping down the slippery ladder of dementia once again.

"Susan, can you get me the thing to stir with?" His ability to retrieve words has become a daily difficulty. He's also challenged getting words past his tongue and out as speech. His face screws up with effort as his tongue twists in his mouth. He starts making less sense and a ten-minute conversation ensues in which he can't get across a complete, sensible thought.

Even though I acknowledge the new decline to friends, it's as though emotionally I'm still clinging to the last plateau, still in denial. As the gulf between these two states grows, I become increasingly irritable and impatient with Bob and with life in general. No one is safe from my grumpiness. My inner critic begins an assault, "You have to be more patient. Look how petty you're becoming! Have some compassion, Susan!" I feel overwhelmed, out of control, and once again a failure as a caregiver.

Relief comes when a friend who hasn't seen Bob for months tells me, "It's shocking to see Bob's decline." This verifies the new reality, which I already know, but haven't consciously accepted. Once that happens, a new bout of grieving surfaces, the critic retreats, the anger subsides and I'm able to be patient and affectionate with my sweet husband once again. Grace returns my joy of life, readying me for the next decline.

For years the busyness of life and the practicalities of survival have cloaked much of my grief, but these are temporary Band-

Aids. Now they're being peeled back, and the rawness of the pain is an open wound that demands all of my attention.

As I sit in Chiesa Santo Spirito, I remember a dream I had years ago. It was night and Bob and I were in a house. Friends were partying in the living room, but Bob and I walked away to a quiet corner. A secret door opened and I saw a darkened lounge with big, overstuffed, comfortable chairs upholstered in neutral gray tones. Someone inside, who I couldn't see, grabbed Bob's arm and started pulling him inside. I grabbed his other arm and struggled to keep him out, knowing if he went in, I'd lose him. I yelled, "No, Bob! Don't go in there!" But he didn't put up a fight. He just let himself be fought over until finally he slipped through my fingers and was pulled inside. The door closed. I slid down the wall in a heap, sobbing, knowing that the love of my life was lost to me forever.

Chapter Two
The Home of the Goddess of the Wind

As we rounded a curve on the 11:20 rapido from Rome
The train left the tracks and leaped into the arms of
Icarus
Cumulus clouds brushed past my window between the
stations of Orion and Cassiopeia
Until we finally stopped at my destination
The Island Behind the Moon

In the spring of 1984, when I was thirty-eight years old, I rented a house on the remote island of Filicudi, Italy. I'd planned to paint, draw, and photograph, as well as to heal from a recent divorce - a divorce that still invaded my dreams both night and day.

Filicudi, whose original name was Phoenicusa, is one of the Aeolian Islands, in a volcanic archipelago in the Tyrrhenian Sea off the northern coast of Sicily. Less than four square miles in size, the island is dry and brush-covered, and in those days had a population of fewer than three hundred hearty folk.

Life on Filicudi wasn't luxurious in the early 1980s. The Greeks had called her 'The Home of the Goddess of the Wind'. Living up to her reputation, the Goddess blew her hot breath across the land, rarely leaving the inhabitants in peace. When she blew mightily the sea washed over the pier, allowing no boats refuge, while the trees defiantly struggled to stay rooted under her rampage.

In this parched terrain, rainwater catchment was a fact of life. The winter rains drained from the roof of my house into a cistern under the living quarters. With no electricity and therefore no pump, I had to master the technique of dropping a wooden bucket into the cistern in just the right way so it filled with water and could be hauled back up. This had to fulfil all my water needs, whether it was washing bed sheets, washing me, or boiling water for tea. I learned to be conservative and grateful for every drop.

The dusty-rose-colored house with its wide veranda was perched on a hill spilling down to the sea. It reminded me of the house my Bohemian grandmother, Francesca, built with her own hands in the 1930's, using wood and other washed-up fragments on Bolinas beach, just north of San Francisco on the California coast. Like her house, there were few sharp angles. All the corners had been softened into voluptuous curves.

It was a thirty-five minute walk from the harbor up a rough volcanic staircase that was often shared with a team of burros transporting goods. There were no cars or motorbikes beyond the harbor. The path led through narrow passageways between houses overgrown with flowering vines. I wore out a pair of Birkenstock sandals in just three months on that vicious, foot-mangling trail.

The house was small and I lived on the veranda when I

didn't need to retreat inside to escape the wind. The kitchen, with only a skylight for a window, was adjacent to a pantry with a precarious ladder that led to two sleeping lofts. But the best room was under the house, with an unobstructed view of the sea. This was the Grotto, the arched-ceiling cave-like room where I slept. There the night was still beyond silence, the black sky shrouded in stars.

A serenade, however, accompanied the sunrise. Rolling up the hill came the braying of donkeys objecting to their loads. Off to the east, the crinkling of a paper sack being breathed in and out by the wind harmonized with the rustle of long grass. A dog barked punctuation. Sheep bleated the new day's gossip.

I spent hours exploring the arid landscape, once inhabited by the people of the Neolithic and Bronze ages. I wandered, sketching and photographing ideas, or just taking in vistas that tickled inspiration. Tumbledown stones with shadowy traces of archaic lettering fed my imagination. I wondered about other people who'd lived here, the Greeks, Romans, and Byzantines, and whether they'd appreciated Filicudi's savage beauty as I did.

The island had three extinct volcanoes, and was full of earthquake ruins overgrown with weeds and vines, and carpeted with flowers gone feral. Those ruins, like my former marriage, dominated my creative vision. As the days wore on, I began to see both from a new perspective.

I was the one who'd left the relationship and I'd somehow thought the dissolution of a fifteen-year marriage would be easier for that. It wasn't. Sometimes the intensity of emotion felt more than I was wired for. I wanted to crawl out of my skin as what-have-I-done, why-did-we-fall-apart, and how-can-love-die questions tore at me day and night.

My ex-husband often suppressed his feelings to the point that I expressed them for both of us. I remember sitting in a restaurant knowing something had been wrong for days and yet he wouldn't admit it. I tried to tiptoe around him because we were in public but the need to ease the tension and understand what was bothering him kidnapped my manners, common sense left me, and I yelled at him. Of course I was very embarrassed, but it got him to talk.

I found it so hard to accept this angry part of myself and yet I wanted to explore and accept it. I saw that my outbursts were preceded by numbness and uncertainty about what I really felt. But when the rush of anger abated, the fog lifted and a new clarity came along with renewed creative energy and joy.

***

Between the healing and deep diving into my psyche, creativity sparked. Poetry has come to me spontaneously over the years, and on the Island Behind the Moon, it thrived. To this day, it comes as a physical sensation I can't ignore. It seems to grow out of my solar plexus and spread into my chest with an energy that galvanizes my attention. That sensation can only be satisfied by holding pen to paper and letting the poem write itself. The poems come, whole or in part, sometimes visually, sometimes as sound. I may be given one line and no other clue until the words spill out onto paper whole and complete and feel right in the mouth when read aloud.

That same creative spark helps me turn sketches into watercolor paintings, layering translucent colors one on top of the other to give a depth not possible with only one hue. This is my usual time-consuming, visionary style. It takes me into a meditative state where time stands still, much as time seemed to do on Filicudi.

Painting and writing are solitary ventures, but too much alone time gets lonely. Needing a balance in order to thrive, I adopted a family. Grazia and Nunzio, a generation older than me, lived just fifteen minutes away. They were always happy to include me at gatherings and to offer a cup of coffee whenever I passed by.

Once, they invited me for a day of labor, teaching me how to bake bread as it had been done on this secluded island for eons. Joining us was their olive-skinned, fiery-eyed daughter-in-law, Pina, and the patriarch, Grandpa Francesco.

Fifty kilos of flour, a half-kilo of yeast, a sack of salt and enough water to hold it all together were dumped into a wooden trough for mixing. Nunzio and Pina kneaded the sticky mass. Grandpa serenaded us with old Sicilian melodies while he shoved bundles of wild *ginestra* into the stone beehive-shaped oven, singing it up to the right temperature. He obviously wasn't too old to enjoy watching Pina's graceful hip movements as she danced the kneading.

Grazia shaped the loaves amid chatter and laughter. My job was to carry them to an inside room and put them to bed between yellow flowered sheets and a rough wool blanket. We sang them a lullaby and left them to rise. But that day they were stubborn and took longer than usual, giving us time for more songs, laughter and banter as Nunzio good-naturedly teased Grazia that it was her fault the loaves were taking their time.

Finally, with sleeves rolled up to reveal gnarly, muscled arms, Francesco slid the loaves into the hot oven on a wooden paddle. Two pizzas to appease the hungry bakers found room in front of the loaves and the door was set in place.

My mother used to say, "The way to a man's heart is through his stomach." That old adage seeped in, and while I had little interest in cooking as a teenager, I quickly followed my gourmet parents' footsteps when I left home. My father's specialties were old-world stews – beef, veal, lamb, or chicken, the soup afloat with plump dumplings. My mother's veal scaloppini and rare roast beef stuck with garlic and rosemary were food for the Gods. Her favorite tastes of asparagus and smoked salmon became mine.

On Sundays my dad often made unusual dishes like eggs with pork chops, with a slice of kidney left in the meat. Though my parents were dismayed when I became vegetarian in my early twenties, their bountiful taste training has stayed with me to this day, and good food and food thoughts permeate my daily life. Baking on Filicudi fit right in.

The bread perfumed the air as the crusts turned golden, taunting our hungry stomachs. When it was done, we let it cool just enough to avoid blistered hands and then broke it up into large pieces returning it to the oven to slowly dry out for the next two days. Then we gorged on fresh herb-scented olive oil smeared pizzas and enough fresh bread to constipate the entire village.

Once dried, the rock hard chunks of *biscotini* were stored in an airtight container to last two months until the next family-bake. Before a meal, enough for each diner would be taken out and covered with water for a few minutes to soften. This wasn't bread-and-butter bread, but bread to dunk in stews and soups, re-inflating and plumping itself in some delightful mix of herbs and broth. My dad would have relished it.

Another day, Grazia asked me to go with her to check on her caper bushes. Filicudi had the largest capers I've ever seen. The shrubs grew wild, scattered over the hills in the searing sun. The buds have to be picked just before the delicate white flower opens. If it blooms, a fruit called a 'caper berry' follows, which is also used in cooking, but isn't as valuable as the caper itself.

Grazia didn't warn me that each bush had an owner. I wandered over to one away from hers to admire the white blossoms. But as I bent to smell the flowers, a disembodied voice bellowed out of the hills: "Leave that bush alone!" Even in what felt a deserted part of this dry land, we were never really alone. After a good laugh, Grazia deftly picked the capers from her numerous bushes and we took them home to pack and layer in sea salt in the way her ancestors had done.

***

Shortly after arriving on Filicudi, I'd noticed how much numbers ruled me. I realized that I ate and slept by the clock. I saw how often I told myself: *Susan, you must work six hours a day. You need eight hours to sleep, two to meditate and two to eat. That leaves six hours to shop, wash, bathe and enjoy this unique place.* I approximated how many calories were in a meal. The pounds showing on a scale could make or break my day. I counted my paintings and figured their value: *three paintings finished, two drawings started, so I still need...* In Filicudi I started to see how absurd I'd become, and that I was treading a sure-fire road to failure.

I'm naturally disciplined, so I was afraid of what would happen if I let go. I'd created my own set of boundaries and I was the policewoman on patrol, shaking her nightstick furiously to make sure those boundaries weren't breached. I'd come to Filicudi to break open these self-imposed walls, but it was like slogging through yesterday's risotto.

In a show of bravado I put my clock away and planned to eat when I was hungry and sleep when I was tired. It wasn't easy. I caught myself watching the sun to see if it was lunchtime yet, and questioning if I'd put in enough hours painting. So much for being a free spirit.

Although my inner voice had been my companion all along, the volume increased. I could hear it without the static of a mind running amok. Or was it that my mind's constant ramblings had taken a rest, and in the silence the knowing came through? It wasn't a disembodied voice. It came from a deeper part of my Being. And magic started to happen.

Four hours into a painting one afternoon, a wave of gratitude welled up in my chest. My inner voice told me to turn off the music, stop painting, sit down and close my eyes. I did, and joy engulfed me. The voice went on: *Go visit Aurora.*

I considered working for another two hours.

Go! said the voice.

Aurora was thirty-seven and had been bedridden for twenty years with a degenerating muscular disease. She smiled broadly when I handed her just-picked yellow roses. We chatted, exchanged news, and sipped dark, sugary espresso. And then I spotted a large peach-colored seashell nestled amongst her books. It was exactly the element I needed for a painting in progress that had been perplexing me with an empty space. There was alchemy in the air. And all I'd done was listen to my intuition.

A few days later I was in the middle of a painting and sensed it needed a dragonfly, but I had only a vague recollection of how they looked. I'd never seen one on the island and my many reference books were gathering dust in my studio back home.

The next morning I was having breakfast on the veranda when a dragonfly landed on a tall weed a foot away. When I made a dash for a pencil, he perched on the stalk as though waiting for my return. As I sketched, he turned again and again so I could draw him from different viewpoints, giving me all the angles I needed. Then we bid each other *arrivederci* and off he flew. I never saw another dragonfly on Filicudi.

***

Most friends who'd heard of this wild, windswept island with a view of three offshore active volcanoes asked if they could visit. I always said yes, but doubted anyone would actually make it to this place my landlord called 'the Island Behind the Moon.' That name was what had sold me on the place. I needed to hide out with myself for a while and face my demons or be consumed by them.

Bob was one of those who'd asked if they could visit. We'd met months before in California, where we'd both left long-term relationships that had run their course. I was living in a basement room rented from friends. As a new single, I'd vowed to keep myself looking presentable, but the morning I ran down to the mailbox with my hair uncombed, wearing rumpled jeans thrown over the thermal underwear I'd slept in the previous night, I wasn't expecting to meet anyone. Then I looked up to see a tall, handsome, grey-haired man in spattered Levi bib-overalls standing on a ladder painting his house.

"Good morning!" he said as he climbed down. "I'm Bob. You're new in the neighbourhood?"

He was friendly and chatty. I wasn't. As soon as I could, I excused myself, saying, "My lunch is on the stove," and disappeared down the gravel driveway muttering something about burned potatoes.

A few hours later there was a knock on the screen door and there he was again, this time shaking me out of my reading reverie, "Hi there!" he chirped, a bit too upbeat for my introverted mood. "I think I have a letter for you that was delivered to my box by mistake. It's addressed to 'Golden Angel'. Would that be you by chance?" I swear I heard him snicker.

I turned beet red as I opened the door to retrieve this letter from a former Italian lover. I didn't offer an explanation.

"Would you like to go out for dinner tonight?" Bob asked.

Nervous about dating again, I made an excuse.

"Well then how about going out for a drink?"

"I don't drink," I explained, uncomfortable at his persistence, and at the same time flattered that this handsome man with a dimpled chin was interested enough to ask me out.

"Order something non-alcoholic then," he countered.

That evening, as we sat in a rustic wooden booth at the most popular eatery in town, Bob told me about the important people in his life: Helen, the brilliant doctor who was his recent ex girlfriend and still his best friend; his quick-tempered ex-wife; his two daughters, Michele and Dawn, both in their twenties, and his one year old grandson, Josh. It was as though a dam wall burst. The words came gushing out, almost washing me away.

I held on tight with a smile and an open mind but I was beginning to feel like a therapist. Finally, at two a.m., the staff told us, "It's time to close".

Saved by the bell! I thought to myself.

Yet Bob had been a perfect gentleman. I took him a bottle of wine a few days later to thank him for gently breaking me back into the dating game. What a huge relief! I felt I could come out of hiding and get on with my life.

And then I left.

My life was moving on, taking me to Turner's watercolor England, where I glided through shallow waters on a canal boat, visited manor houses, and tramped along misty waterway paths. From England I went on to Florence to study Italian. I'd had a love affair with Italy and all things Italian since high school and my dream was to live in Italy. Little did I know the Universe had other plans.

I gave Bob a call when I got back to the States and we met for dinner. After our first date when his emotional dam broke and he clearly needed a listener, I found on the second meeting a sincere, down to earth man who put me at ease and was interested in what I had to say. He knew how to have a conversation, and with his easy, mellow ways and abundant sense of humor, I could see he was a rarity. My radar, however, told me he was only interested in me as a friend and I wasn't ready to get back into a relationship. When I called again as he'd asked me to, and left a message, he didn't call back. I had no way of knowing he never got that message.

Weeks later, by chance, I struck up a conversation with a woman in a cafe, and something she said made me realise I was talking to Bob's ex.

"We have a mutual friend - Bob Behrens," I said.

"Then you must be Susan, the artist? He's always talking about you!"

"Well, if he talks about me, then why doesn't he call?"

"Bob's very shy. And he's worried about your age difference," said Helen. "You need to call him."

And so I did, and again he invited me for dinner. That night, somewhere between the salad and main course, with our eyes expressing more than our words, I felt a switch flip in my psyche and my body. Suddenly, I wanted this man. He must have sensed it. When he took my hand, we were playing a completely different game. Later, after he drove me back to where I was parked, we were like magnets, hardly able to pull ourselves apart. I couldn't get my van started because he'd commandeered my hands. The windows steamed up as we worked ourselves into a frenzied corner of passion, but there was no way out. I was staying with my parents and he had his daughters living with him. A hotel room seemed tacky.

The next night desire overthrew discretion and he invited me to stay. For five days we couldn't get enough of each other. And then I left for Filicudi.

I'd suggested Bob come for the last week of my stay on the island so I'd have the time I needed to sort myself out, and to paint and write before he arrived. I'd told him I'd take him to all my favorite places in Italy. But I doubted he'd make it. Filicudi wasn't easily accessible and this was a man who'd only traveled to Canada for skiing and Mexico for Club Med.

The mail was notoriously slow in that part of Italy. I went to the post office almost daily, but after a month I was beginning to have doubts Bob would write, let alone visit. In self-defense, I tried to push away thoughts of him, but the sweetness of our short time together lingered.

And all the while I was pouring my heart out to him in multi-page letters with wildflowers affixed to a corner, sharing my deepest and most vulnerable parts, exposing what I was learning about myself in those weeks of self-imposed exile and healing. Had I shown too much?

At the pinnacle of this anxiety, and five weeks into my retreat, there was a *Sciopero* on the island, one of those infamous Italian strikes. Sixteen citizens, two dogs and three placards turned the boats away from Porto Pecorini for the second day in a row. No tourists, no produce, no mail, no outside influence infiltrated Filicudi. And yet outside influence was what the strike was about. The locals looked longingly at the night lights on nearby Salina and Lipari. The anticipation of electric power, phones, and roads brought them to the port twice a day, hoping someone would listen.

The three dozen renegades and runaways who came here to escape their secret shadows wanted to keep Filicudi as it was – a distant oasis wearing the tattered clothing of the past. But now the shop shelves stood empty, echoing the pleas carried across the sea. "Is anybody listening?"

All through this drama the Goddess toyed with us, blowing gale force through the night, making sleep impossible. I lay in the dark feeling her tirade, diving deeper under my covers and wondering if my white knight would come to claim me.

The next day the grapevine relayed up the hill, *"Suzanna c'e' qualche cosa alla posta!"* I had mail. But the muse had me in her hold, so I continued to paint, brushing back the urge to check out what might be waiting, afraid of disappointment.

It was afternoon before the muse loosened her grip. I cleaned my brushes and stumbled bleary-eyed down the hill with several cards to drop in the letterbox. I'd missed the open hours and didn't even hope for a reprieve, given what everyone had been through in recent days.

Whistling a catchy tune, the postman was tending his garden

alongside the office, which doubled as his home. "Is it true I have mail? If so, I'll come back first thing in the morning."

"No, no Signora!" With an uncustomary flourish, he unlocked the door and handed me my precious booty.

Mail was my only contact with the outside world. It was a drug and I was addicted. My heart started to pound when I saw unfamiliar writing on an envelope. I had my first letter and a package from Bob.

I tried not to grin too wildly as I scampered off to find a quiet rock overlooking the sea where I could open my treasures and devour the contents. A photo of Bob fell out from the pages and relief washed over me when I read that he'd just applied for his first passport and was shopping for a backpack. The letter made me cry and smile and giggle. I read it twice.

The package contained a cassette tape. That night, I took it to the Grotto, lit candles and a sandalwood incense stick, snuggled under my covers and pressed 'play'. His deep, sexy voice left me reeling, almost dizzy with delight, followed by gut-wrenching fear.

Bob was a traveling salesman, selling drapes and mini blinds. He had an aging, yellow Cadillac with a good sound system for road trips, which had been a birthday present from his ex-girlfriend, Helen, the woman who'd convinced me to make that call. She was a woman who knew very well that a Taurus needs his comforts. On the tape, Bob told me he'd suddenly started to notice all the love songs playing on the radio, songs he'd been deaf to before. He'd had a jack installed in the car so he could plug his tape recorder into it, record songs that spoke to him, and then add his comments to me. By the end of the tape it was obvious this man was in love, and I was the love object.

I didn't know what to think. I was happy and excited, but what did I really feel about him after only five days of intense connection and as many weeks of imagination gone wild? I was scared. *What in Hell had I gotten myself into?*

I attached the photo to the wall by my painting table. Boberto, as I'd taken to calling him, reminded me of a teddy bear, and I wanted to crawl through the emulsion and wrap my arms around him. I listened to his tape till I could almost recite his words verbatim, captivated by his playful, baritone voice. But I was a ball of confused emotions: elated that this handsome man wanted me, afraid of letting him down, and still raw from self-discovery and from divorce.

I had a month remaining to do what I'd come to the island to do, and hopefully, I could stay present while I tried to figure things out. But time was running away with me. I'd have to work feverishly to get my paintings done before he arrived. And I still hadn't cracked the big life questions like *Who am I?* and *What's it all about, Alfie?*

***

One day, word was relayed up the hill through cupped hands, "*Suzaaannna! Telegrammma!*" I rushed down. Bob had written that he'd call the only telephone in the village in nine days time at four o'clock in the afternoon.

There was often a long line of people waiting to use the solitary phone. It was a half hour walk from my house and I arrived early, antsy, unable to sit still. *Stai tranquilla*! – the

Italian command to be calm - wasn't working, no matter how many times or how loudly it was directed at me.

The call was late, adding to my tension. Then a bad connection made it necessary to shout into the receiver so nearly the whole village was privy to our conversation. Between sizzles of static, Bob told me he'd gotten his ticket and was still shopping for a backpack. I couldn't stop smiling.

"There are a few obstacles though." He paused. "I'll probably lose my job over this. My boss refuses to give me time off. And looks like I'll have to borrow some money from Helen. I don't care. I can't wait to hold you again."

As he told me about his itinerary, Bob didn't know he couldn't have devised a better plan to capture my heart. The idea that a man would travel halfway around the world, possibly losing his job to find me, was seductive.

However, as the reality of his arrival drew near, it collided with my romantic notions. I began to feel more cautious and less sure of myself. Still grappling with the end of one relationship, I wasn't sure I was ready to dive into another.

Seeing how nervous I was, my women friends hatched a plan to accompany me to the ferry. We'd be a royal entourage greeting the Prince as he disembarked, and hopefully waylaying Enrico, the village leper and Filicudi's self-appointed greeting committee. Enrico had been dramatically disfigured by the disease, but he always dressed impeccably in slacks, jacket, and tie. He derived great pleasure from thrusting out his hand with its missing fingers to unsuspecting travelers. He welcomed them heartily with a wide smile, but I was sure inside he was having a great belly laugh as he watched their faces register his missing nose and ears.

Slowly, the white inter-island ferry pulled up to the dock. My stomach lurched as the gangway was set in place and passengers began disembarking. My gaggle of friends were nearly as tense as I was. My fingernails pressed into my hands while one woman paced and another one twisted her hair. They were there to support me, but I suspected they were also very curious to meet this man who'd come halfway around the world to find me.

We scrutinized the passengers carefully. "Is that him?" someone would point and ask.

"I'm not sure," I'd stammer. "I haven't seen him for three months."

But it soon became clear that none of these men was 'him'. As the dock emptied, my stomach knotted and a sinking feeling settled into my solar plexus. Thoughts buzzed through my mind, all knocking into each other. *Is he alright? What if he's ill? Maybe he missed the boat. Maybe he changed his mind.* This last one grew louder and louder.

My friends tried to buoy me up. "He most likely missed the connection. Or got the wrong directions. Few people speak English on Sicily." Reading the disappointment on my face, they assured me he'd arrive the next day.

***

I awoke to a splendid day with a scattering of puffy white clouds to break up the Mediterranean blue, but I felt dazed. My mind was whirring at record speed, making it difficult to focus.

I kept telling myself *He might not be on this boat either. And that will still be alright*, as though repeating this mantra would keep disappointment away. The truth was, I was scared. Five romantic days, then three months apart with only a tape, a few letters and telegrams, and a couple of phone calls wasn't much to go on. I hadn't a clue how I really felt about Bob. I still didn't trust my emotions. And now, we'd be together continuously for three and a half weeks. What if my anger popped up like an uninvited dinner guest? Or maybe we'd just have a vacation fling and that would be all? My mind was jabbing me in all my most tender places.

The previous day's scene repeated itself, except that this time I had no entourage; I was a welcoming committee of one. Enrico was at his station as the ferry docked, the gangway was lowered and secured, and my heart pounded harder with each disembarking passenger.

The human stream became a trickle. *I might not be up to this*, I thought, my breath catching in my throat. Then, finally, the very last passenger walked down the gangplank: a tall curly-gray-haired man in blue jeans and a tee shirt sporting a very large red backpack.

Oh shit! What do I do now? I was shaking and excited, happy and relieved. Tears streaked down my cheeks.

We hugged as if we'd just discovered each other after being shipwrecked on opposite ends of a deserted island. "You're as beautiful as I remembered," he whispered, and three months melted away, taking with them my fears and apprehensions. I remembered why I wanted the look of him, the smell of him near.

Up we climbed, single file along the narrow path to my castle on the mountainside, stopping to catch our breath now and then and take in the panorama. That day smoke lazily curled up from the volcano on neighboring Vulcano while Sicily's Mt. Etna lay quietly in the distance.

Once at the house, we were hesitant with each other, both unsure of ourselves as we talked about his journey and my time on Filicudi. I was nervously flitting about, showing him the house, when we suddenly collided into a long embrace punctuated by gentle kisses. The tension melted and we melded. Our clothes pooled on the floor and I took him by the hand to my whitewashed Grotto below for marathon lovemaking that deepened our connection psychically as well as physically.

***

Over the next five days Filicudi's witchcraft spun a web of love and magic around us. We visited the ruins that had inspired my paintings. I introduced him to friends who pulled me aside, one by one, to tell me what a truly nice man he was. We hiked the hills and I tricked Bob into smelling the caper flowers, knowing the disembodied voice would shout, "Keep away!" and leave me roaring with laughter. We sat under the stars on moonless nights, marveling at the vast, star-strewn sky. And we picnicked on the pebbled beach, eating bread with slabs of aromatic pecorino cheese, and sweet blood oranges, and sipping red wine until it was time for a dip.

I've never been comfortable in water, but Bob was like a fish.

As I sat on the shore watching his head bob beyond the waves, I could feel his joy in being one with the power of Neptune. It was a vicarious thrill watching him become amphibious. "I grew up at the beach," he told me later. "I think I learned to swim before I learned to walk!"

Through it all, Bob was easy to be with, mellow, and interested in everything. We never lacked for things to talk about. The only time we lapsed into a mutual silence was to communicate on a different level. Neither of us felt as if this was a new relationship. It felt as if we'd been reunited.

***

It wasn't easy for me to say farewell to Filicudi. I went from room to veranda to room, touching a wall, a table, a candle, a chair, a cushion, and releasing them from my emotional grip. The house on the hill had been a sanctuary where I found myself again and became more comfortable in my own skin. I felt realigned, and I understood just how important it is for me to have solitude and to recognise that need when it arises.

Our time in the house was over and the next tenants were ready to move in. Bob helped me pack my paintings and accompanied me as I said goodbye to all the people who'd touched my life. Grazia and I held each other and wept, knowing we'd never see each other again. But I was leaving the Island Behind the Moon with a burgeoning new love, and although we didn't know it yet, the ride of our lives was in the offing.

Chapter Three
Favorite Places

Until one is committed, there is hesitancy,
the chance to draw back,
always ineffectiveness.
Concerning all acts of initiative
there is one elementary truth
the ignorance of which kills countless ideas and endless plans.
That the moment one definitely commits oneself,
then Providence moves too.
All sorts of things occur to help one
that would never otherwise have occurred.
A whole stream of events issues from the decision,
raising in one's favor all manner of unforeseen incidents
and meetings and material assistance,
which no man could have dreamed would come his way.
Whatever you can do or dream you can,
begin it.
Boldness has genius, power, and magic in it.

-W.H. Murray from *The Scottish Himalayan Expedition*

The sun illuminated the dusky blue sky with smears of pink and orange before it peeked over the horizon as we held each other on the deck of a Naples-bound ferry. Churning through a sapphire sea, we'd been famished for each other and tried to sleep in the same narrow berth in our windowless cabin. Little sleep and a lot of laughter came in those hot, cramped quarters; being close was more nourishing than food or rest. Our batteries, charged on love and lust chemicals, made us feel intensely alive.

We brushed Naples aside, hopping the next train to Florence for our second stop on the 'Susan's Taste of Italy' tour. By mid-afternoon we were checking into a *pensione* near the famous white, green, and pink marble-faced *Duomo*, the cathedral that dominates the cityscape.

I'd been enamored with this majestic white lily of a city with food fit for the Medici from my first visit in 1976. I'd returned several times, and finally studied Italian there in 1983 while immersing myself again and again in the masterpieces of art and architecture. Michelangelo, Donatello, Di Vinci, Bernini, Botticelli, and Fra Filippo Lippi were some of my favorite Renaissance artists represented there. This was art history in the flesh.

Once on the streets, I showed Bob the *Firenze* I knew and loved. I took him down narrow, cobblestoned alleyways, popping out into bustling squares with flower sellers and well-dressed Italians going about their daily lives. Children screeched their delight as their voices bounced off walls their ancestors had built centuries before.

A morning ritual developed with the concierge of our *pensione*. She'd knock on our door. "You're wasting your time! *Firenze* is out there waiting for you! *Andate!*" she'd chide, and with muffled laughter, Bob would call out, "We'll get an earlier start tomorrow." Giggling, we'd dive back under the covers for round two. The Renaissance would have to wait.

***

On the other side of the Arno, the river that cuts a wide swathe through the city, we wound our way up the steep labyrinth of streets to San Miniato al Monte, a Romanesque church started in the 11th century. With a stunning panorama overlooking the city and reaching beyond the medieval city walls, it was not only inviting inside, but spellbinding outside. Hours seeped by in the quiet of those hills, and by the time we made our way back to the other side of the river, we were famished.

The famous gelateria, Vivoli's, solved that problem. But it was a difficult decision between *stracciatella, zabaglione*, and *cioccolato all'arancio* – orange-laced chocolate so dark it was almost black. We returned the next day for *lampone, caffe*, and *nocciola,* not feeling the slightest bit guilty for our decadent mix of raspberry, coffee and hazelnut under a swirl of whipped cream.

Strolling along the Arno, we saw single rowers and teams practicing for upcoming races, the sound of their oars dipping and slicing through the water, hypnotizing us to stay and watch. Behind us, the piazza of the Uffizi Gallery, housed in a sixteenth-century palace, was a circus of activity with vendors selling trinkets and art reproductions, and caricature artists with rainbow displays of pastels and finished drawings calling out to attract customers.

After this full day of sightseeing we discovered we both relished people-watching. Sipping *Spritz Aperol*, the famous bitter orange cocktail topped with bubbly Prosecco, in Piazza Signoria, we marveled at people marveling at the Renaissance sculpture in the square. Bob noticed things I'd never paid attention to. "See how that woman in red walks on the insides of her shoes? She's probably insecure." And "That man over there chews his lip while he reads. I'll bet he's a worrier." And "Look how open with wonder that young girl's face is." While I taught him about art, he was teaching me to read people.

He told me that in third grade he'd been dragged to the front of the classroom, held by the scruff of the neck and rebuked by the teacher for chronic daydreaming. Held back a grade while his peers moved on, he'd been ridiculed at recess for being stupid. This strangled any trust he might have had of kids his own age, and so he'd become a loner, honing his observation skills to better understand who was friend and who was foe. Now, these observations were automatic to him and fascinating to me.

The next morning we entered the Uffizi Art Gallery hand in hand. This temple of Italian masterpieces was sacred territory to me, housing paintings that stirred my deepest recesses, rekindling and feeding my creative cauldron. Bob sensed how important a place this was to me. With bowed heads we passed through the portal, speaking in hushed tones or moving along in silence.

Sandro Botticelli's large painting, 'Spring', with its delicate, transparent fabrics blowing in a breeze always took my breath away no matter how many times I gazed at it. Botticelli painted hands and feet so sensually I wanted to crawl into the paintings and nuzzle them. This kind of place was my church, my connection to the Divine. Sensing this, Bob teared up from the sheer majesty of this world. He, too, connected to the creative spirit here, even though he had no words for it.

The next day, in another of my favorite spots in Florence, the cathedral of Santa Croce, I showed him the famous Giotto frescos. These paintings are less refined than many we'd seen at the Uffizi but still they have something special. Bob asked, "Why are they so historically important and yet so naive?"

"Giotto was the first artist in a thousand years to grapple with linear perspective. Before him, everyone painted flat, one-dimensional images. So he ended up being one of the most important painters of the fourteenth century. He unknowingly started The Renaissance – though it wouldn't be in full swing for another seventy years."

Bob soaked this all in, thirsty for new ideas and for anything that touched him deeply. He loved Shakespeare and classical music, but he knew little of art. He felt alive with new possibilities. "I've waited fifty-two years for this," he whispered in the hush of the cathedral. "And for you."

Those first weeks together were so easy. "It's as though we were treading water waiting for this reunion," he breathed in my ear, his arms encircling me as we watched the sunset from the Ponte Vecchio, the old bridge spanning the River Arno.

At twilight, this quintessential Florentine landmark became patchworked with colorful cloths spread with handicrafts from all over the world. Like a Middle Eastern bazaar, it was a riot of color and a pastiche of characters, some pierced and tattooed, some in traditional costumes from faraway places, all haggling and selling until late into the evening. Although we didn't yet know it, this tapestry was a premonition of what would transpire for us in the next few years.

We wandered the narrow streets on our last day, getting lost in the labyrinth of the five-hundred-year-old *palazzi* that affirmed the power and wealth of this great city. Strolling along opposite the *Duomo*, we fell into conversation about our return to the States.

"I guess I'll have to stay with my parents again while I find a place to live," I said. "It isn't easy to go back home when you're an adult."

"Why don't you move in with me?"

My heart stopped mid beat. *Does he mean move IN with him, as in live together? Or does he mean move in until I find a place of my own?*" I was too shy to ask.

"You're the love of my life, Susan! Life's too short to mess around."

I pondered this for a few more blocks, then threw my arms around his neck and squealed, "Yes, yes, yes!"

***

Cinque Terre is a string of five rainbow-colored villages on the rugged west coast of Liguria, northwest of Florence. There were no roads between these hamlets, only railway tracks and paths. The train snaked us through the dark-and-light of tunnels and stations with only a few tantalizing glimpses of the coast below until we disembarked in the postcard-perfect village of Vernazza, with its small boat harbor and house-encrusted hills rising sharply in a U shape around the center. The smell of the salt air instantly relaxed any travel tension.

A maze of wooden fishing boats lay scattered on the broad launch ramp. Some sported fat, languid house cats sleeping on colorful canvas boat covers. Vernazza was a feline-friendly town with cats to pet and play with, cats curled together in planters, and cats that crawled into our laps for a snuggle. They were oblivious to the waves crashing over the seawall that sent unsuspecting tourists scattering for dry land.

We found a room halfway up steep winding stairs leading to a castle perched on the edge of a cliff where the sea collided with the wall below. "Come, my love! See the royal jewels set before us, hear the royal orchestra," Bob said as he guided me over to the small window in our room. It opened out to the setting sun, casting golden ripples on the sea.

That evening, after dining on *risotto pescadore*, a dish of creamy rice and just caught seafood, we heard singing and the strum of guitar and mandolin. The strings beckoned us, leading us through a narrow maze of passageways. Curiosity pulled us up a short flight of stairs and through an archway to a small café where two musicians and eight male singers belted out songs woven from life's joys and sorrows .

We soaked in the music with a glass of *Sciacchetra*, Cinque

Terre's famed dessert wine, made rich and dense by hanging grapes to dry and concentrate their juices. Each autumn the whole of Vernazza is festooned with bunches of these grapes in dark nooks and crannies, perfuming the air with fermentation.

We kissed unabashedly and clinked our glasses. "To you, Suz, my special delivery at the mail box. And to our good fortune." Our eyes locked in deep embrace, eliciting approving smiles from the musicians and diners around us.

During hot sunny days we hiked between the villages along narrow paths etched between crowded terraces of wine grapes and olives. After centuries of grueling labor, no horizontal patch of land had been left uncultivated and only the most steeply vertical remained intact. We met few people and revelled in the silence.

I took a photo of my handsome, sweet man, shirtless in khaki pants, sitting in a field of perfumed white wildflowers just outside the hilltop town of Corniglia. This photo was to make its way to our future home, reminding us of our heady beginnings. Years later I'd look at and be transported, for a few moments, away from Alz world.

After descending the steep zigzag of nearly four hundred stairs on the other side of town we made our way to the beach for a refreshing swim before moving on to Manarola, perhaps the oldest of the five villages, where the cornerstone of the church dates from the fourteenth century. Ravenous, we found a small outdoor café on the entrance to the boat ramp. A warren of impossibly quaint, pastel-colored houses jutted up the hillside around us. As we supped on fettuccini with dill-brushed smoked salmon simmered in a splash of white wine, we felt like we were in an over-the-top romantic comedy.

At the last of the villages, Riomaggiore, we strolled the winding cliffside *Via dell'Amore*, or Lover's Walk, tossing a rainbow of just-picked wild flowers into the crashing waves below. Watching them swirl in the opalescent sea foam, we shouted, "To life and love!" in a spontaneous ceremony to our heart connection. Bob winked and faked a yawn, "Isn't it time for a nap?"

It was. Vernazza and our seaview room was only a ten-minute train ride away.

***

Our time in Italy was coming to a close and I still had my favorite city, *La Serenissima*, 'The Most Serene Republic of Venice' to show my new man. We arrived late in the morning, popping out of the Santa Lucia train station into a dream-like setting. Venice's jewels glinted off the water, captivating us instantly. After dropping our bags at a *locanda* near Piazza San Stefano, we began the rambling exploration I so love in Venice. I always have a map tucked away in my bag but rarely use it since most maps of Venice are useless. Getting lost is an everyday occurrence and half the enjoyment. We surrendered to the muse.

It was love at first sight for Bob, as it had been for me when I first came, eight years before. We lost ourselves among small *sotto portico* passageways that took us under houses, through narrow lanes, and canal-side walkways, often popping us out onto thriving squares full of produce sellers, children playing, and grandmas sitting on wooden benches catching up with the local gossip, perfect places to stop at an outdoor café for a strong, dark espresso.

The canals fascinated us. We rode *vaporetti*, the often-crowded public boats, hopping on and off as whim dictated to explore some enticement glimpsed from the railing as the boat approached a dock. We were spellbound by alleyways so narrow we had to walk single file, fragments of thousand-year-old symbols incorporated into more modern walls, and a profusion of ever-changing water reflections.

We asked a passerby to photograph us on the small San Polo Bridge. With arms wrapped around each other, my head on his shoulder, we beamed a smile into the camera. Twenty-two years later, on our final trip to Italy together, we'd take that photo with us, find the bridge after days of searching, and do a repeat performance, wondering how we could have aged so much when we felt so young inside and our love was still thriving.

Holding hands as we drifted to sleep on our last night in Venice, the sound of singing pulled us back to consciousness. Dressing quickly, we rushed downstairs and out into the midnight air, blindly following the siren call, and finally emerged into a moonlit Piazza San Marco, the most famous Piazza of them all, to find a choral group belting out their delight. Sitting on a small step, arms around each other, soaking in the music, the stars, and the magic of Venice, we were filled with gratitude to be in this extraordinary city, basking in the glow of new love.

When the musicians finally moved on, singing their way back to their hotel, we meandered back to ours with visions of the glittering gold Basilica and the four bronze horses standing guard high above the square accompanying our return.

**

We had a perfect beginning, falling in love in the most romantic of lands without pressure or hindrance. We saw only the good and beautiful in each other and love flourished. But the time finally came to return to the real world, to try on our new life together and see how it fit back in the States, back in the realm of work and taxes, friends and family, and the trials and tribulations of everyday life. And what trials those were to become!

Chapter Four
Where Did You Go?

Reality
Sanity
What is real?
What is accurate?
The line blurs
There can only be
One Truth
And it absolutely cannot be contained
Within a thought

Two and a half decades later, the reverie of our beginnings holds me captive as I stroll along Florence's Arno River on this, my first respite trip away from Bob. It feels as though I've come full circle. Twenty-six years ago I'd been in Italy grieving the loss of one relationship while a new one was gestating. And now I'm grieving the loss of that love to Alzheimer's. I know a fresh way of being has to evolve, but I feel totally blind to what that freshness will be and what it might bring. I remind myself that in order for something to be born, something else must die, just as the act of creating a painting destroys the pure white void of canvas or paper.

I've been part of a couple nearly all my adult life. And my

couplings have been mostly unconventional, full-on working together connections as opposed to working separately eight or more hours a day. But perhaps this is the time for me to learn to be on my own. In many ways it's already happened, since I now have all the responsibilities Bob and I used to share, plus the responsibility of his care.

The business that has supported us for more than a decade evolved organically, starting with one employee and burgeoning into thirty. It was Bob who interfaced with our twenty craftsmen, driving up to their village several times a week. He was my back-up and support, taking care of the maintenance of machines and vehicles, doing all the driving, and leaving me to design our creations and take care of correspondence and organization. When I cooked, he cleaned up. Slowly, as the disease has progressed and he can no longer do his work, I've assimilated it or found others to fill in.

As my workload increases I have the added responsibility of caring for a man who often feels like a familiar stranger with the needs of a child, a man unable to take care of himself as his hold on language and body control slips away. My ears, always attuned to where he is and what he's doing in order to to keep him safe, are also inundated with his brain-numbing, repetitive questioning. "What's on the schedule for today?" he asks for the tenth time in an hour. It's a challenge to focus on what's before me.

It's been my intention since he was first diagnosed with Alzheimer's to keep Bob with me as long as possible and to care for him in a way that he can thrive as fully as possible given his condition. Our great love continually feeds this strong resolve. But while the intention is firm, I often feel I fall short of being a good caregiver. I seem to tumble off the patience wagon more often than is comfortable and am forever straining to pull myself back on, vowing to be better but not able to fully realize that desire.

Sometimes I watch as my body and psyche shut down. It can happen gradually or swiftly. There's a physical reaction, often centered in the solar plexus, as well as an emotional retreat that can be triggered by something as innocuous as Bob staring at me while I cook.

It's dinnertime. We're in our small kitchen. "What's for dinner?" Bob asks for the third time.

"Pasta with smoked tuna and an arugula salad with sun-dried tomatoes." I'm a frantic, focused cook, moving quickly around the kitchen with no time to wash up as I go.

"What's for dinner?"

"Pasta and salad," I say with strained patience. The smell of sautéed garlic and onions fills the room. I try to distract Bob with jobs like setting the table or washing whatever I've already thrown in the sink or piled up on the counter.

"What's for dinner?"

"We're having a yummy pasta and a crisp green salad." I try to brighten my answer and my resolve to be patient as I pour white wine into the sauce, but in reality it's better to repeat the same answer. I secretly try to dirty as many items as possible to keep him busy, but as soon as he's finished he stands off to the side, just on the edge of my peripheral vision, almost at military attention, and watches my every move.

"What's for dinner?"

Logically, I know there's no harm in this watching or questioning. Logically, I know he's bored and has nothing else to do and I'm his only entertainment. Logically, I know this has nothing to do with me. But emotionally it drives me mad. It triggers a reaction I'm not proud of - shutting down and becoming crisp cold. I watch this happen and feel powerless to stop it. It's not until my brain chemicals subside and the gate of warmth opens that I can really be with him again, friendly and affectionate.

I've studied these shutdowns, trying to figure out a way out of them, a way of being more compassionate with my husband. Sometimes they come upon me for no special reason and I watch myself retreat inside a suit of armor. The harder I struggle, the more locked-in and distant I become. It feels like I reach a point where I've had enough and I just can't give anymore.

I've realized 'the only way out is through' and the only thing to do is to be as aware as possible of what's truly going on. It seems to me that this awareness holds the key to healing. I also see the need to have compassion for myself and for what I'm endeavoring to do. Awareness and self-patience don't come easily.

I don't know if there is ever one answer to these episodes, or if each one has to be looked at anew, but it's through self-awareness and gentleness that I come to understand that distancing myself emotionally from Bob is a way to catch my breath, to have a reprieve from the constant questions and comments that are so intellectually numbing, to have a sense of space when he hovers around me.

The Bob I fell in love with was a generous man who cared about other people. He was the kind of man the checker in the grocery store would pour his or her heart out to while ringing up the groceries. When a friend needed something fixed, Bob would offer to do it. But now that the connection with others is lost, his generosity of spirit has retreated. He's lost the ability to problem solve, so fixing things is out. And he can't hold onto a story well enough to be a good listener, so he just stays quiet.

Bob adored me. He showed his appreciation of what we shared by his words and actions on a daily basis, building me tables and shelves to set up a painting studio, and willingly helping around the house.

One time I had an idea for a plant stand utilizing an old pair of Bob's striped ski pants He enthusiastically grabbed hold of the idea and spent a few hours at his workbench building the inner wooden structure. The ski pants had been a joke between us because they were so garish and out of style. When he put the stand together he surprised me with a pair of his well-worn shoes below the pant legs so the finished piece looked like a standing man from the waist down. The plant stood on a board inserted in the top of the pants to make a table. This sentinel stood in our hallway, where it brought a lot of laughter. Bob even made comments to it when he entered the house, as though it had its own personality.

While Bob still occasionally tells me he loves me, it's with a hint of rote and habit, as though he knows he should say this. Or perhaps there's a temporary clearing in his mind and so he feels it in that moment. I just know I feel desperately, cloyingly needed by Bob for his survival, while the unconditional love of a husband for his wife has evaporated.

Sadly, Alzheimer's has taken the give and take that's normal and restorative in a relationship and made it heavily lopsided. It's robbed Bob of his sense of 'the other' or the importance of the other. He seems to be in survival mode at all times, always on the lookout for who might be trying to take advantage of him.

The one time Bob seems to truly care about something other than himself is when he comes in contact with a dog or a cat. Then he's really there, stroking the animal, cooing to it, acting in a way he no longer can with humans.

Sometimes I think, *Whoever you are in my husband's body, go away! I want my Sweet Wonderful Man back!* At the same time, I feel strongly that it's my turn to give back to my beloved. He's always been supportive of my crazy ideas, supportive of how I function in the world. He went along with my dream to take off on a four-month trip to Southeast Asia, putting all our possessions in storage, after a particularly difficult year. He encouraged plans for travel. And he was happy to live in another country and learn another language, embracing my idea as his own.

Bob essentially jumped on my dream wagon, took hold of the reins, steered and protected me, yelling, "Yahoo! Let's go for a ride!" He was my safety net. And now I'm his.

Though we've lived a colorful, inspiring life together, for which I'm eternally grateful, that doesn't assuage the huge loss of having my soulmate disappear piece-by-piece right before my eyes. It's profound torture.

Chapter Five
Down the Rabbit Hole

The pain of separation creeps in on little cat feet
Scrambling thought waves
Tearing open joyousness
Leaving discarded shards at my feet
It sits on my shoulder
With the reminder that bliss
Is not won in a lottery
Or found in a lost wallet belonging to someone else
No other human no matter how elevated
Can take our hand and lead us out of separation
It's a solo flight
Through pain and fear
Into Oneness

Dwarfed by Pelton wheels and other rusted mining equipment in the lobby of the American Victorian Museum, I awaited my entrance cue. I was wearing the layered lace, sea-foam green dress I'd purchased in London ten months earlier and kept hidden for this occasion.

Ivan Najera strummed the refrain from John Denver's 'Annie's Song' on his guitar in this old Gold Rush foundry, a veritable institution in Nevada City and a perfect place for a wedding.

He sang, "You fill up my senses, like a night in the forest,"

Eighty guests turned, their eyes focused on me as I entered the room clutching my bouquet of white roses and lilies and trying not to shake.

"Like the mountains in spring time, like a walk in the rain,"

Tears of joy streamed down my face.

"Like a storm in the desert, like a sleepy blue ocean,"

Bob stood at the front of the hall, gallant and handsome in a gray tweed jacket shot with peach, the same peach as his silk shirt and tie.

"You fill up my senses, come fill me again,"

Magnetically, his smile pulled me towards him. He was my tether. Crying through my grin, I was afraid to look directly at anyone for fear of totally losing control.

"Come let me love you, let me give my life to you,"

This was a bad idea! Don't listen to the words -This song always does me in!

"Let me drown in your laughter, let me die in your arms,"

Tears were streaming down both our faces as Ivan belted out the last lines of 'our song',

"Let me lay down beside you, let me always be with you,

Come let me love you, come love me again."

There wasn't a dry eye in the house and we hadn't even

begun spluttering out our carefully written vows to one another, vows that came from two hearts meeting and melding, sharing the love of a lifetime.

***

We'd been living together for nearly a year in Bob's house in Auburn, California, and were perfectly contented. We'd talked easily about anything and everything except one subject. We'd skirted around it, treading carefully as though it were Pandora's Box and the slightest bump would snap it open and bring the wrath of God upon us.

In the deep of night when sleep was elusive I'd wonder how Bob felt about marriage. *Does he ever want to take the plunge again? Or has he sworn it off after his first experience?*

Discomfort built. The elephant in the room kept getting bigger, feeding on our blaring silence. Friends and family nagged me, wanting to know if-when-where-how. I finally worked up the courage to broach the subject one starry night in the hot tub on the deck outside our bedroom. As nonchalantly as possible, I asked, "So, what do you think about marriage?"

My white knight nearly choked on the sip of wine he was taking. He sputtered, clearly surprised. I assured him I wasn't proposing, only wanting to know what he felt since we seemed to dance around the subject, never landing in its center.

We talked openly and honestly that night. He told me that marriage was an important commitment to him, one that he didn't take lightly. He didn't know if he wanted to remarry since he'd already had kids and didn't want more. The possibility of us tying the knot wasn't discussed. I was satisfied with our discussion and thought that was the end of it until we were sitting in a Nevada City café a month later. Bob lifted his glass to me and said, "Why don't we get married when we meet in London next month?"

I was the one choking this time.

As romantic as it sounded, after a few weeks deliberation we decided not to run off and get married in a foreign country, but to be surrounded by friends and loved ones. Ours was a love to share.

We planned, cooked, and decorated, doing most of the work ourselves, seeing this celebration as a gift to our friends and family as well as a tribute to our love.

***

Lynn, the non-denominational minister, and our two best friends, Helen and Jan, were there to steady us as well as to be official witnesses. I liked to joke that Bob's best man was a woman, the same Helen who'd propelled us together two years before and would be an integral part of our lives for years to come. Jan had been my closest friend for a decade. We'd gone through each other's divorces, always there with space for the other to talk or vent or cry.

Standing on an easel framed in gold was 'Soul Mates', a visionary watercolor painting I'd done of us in various incarnations from cave couple to ancient Egyptians to Samurai and wife. Prints of it had been attached to our wedding invitations. Now a forest of white calla lilies, casually tossed in tall, clear glass vases, surrounded it. They seemed to be craning their long necks for a better view of the proceedings.

Lynn called our closest loved ones up to the front of the room to form a circle around us. Our rings, with gold images of our faces merging, were passed around the circle for each person to bless as they cradled them in their hands and acknowledged us as a couple. Our guests weren't mere witnesses; they were participants in this celebration. It was a reminder to other couples of the love that had brought them together and an inspiration to the singles that anything is possible at any time in life.

The room was charged with warmth, energy and love as we croaked our vows out to one another, barely able to speak through tears of joy and elation. When we kissed life into our marriage, a cheer rose up. As we walked down the aisle, I didn't know who was beaming more, our guests or us.

With the official ceremony over and the papers signed and dated, March 22, 1986, we walked proudly out to the street in a shower of rice to where a white satin-bedecked wedding carriage with a huge, equally white Clydesdale horse waited to take us on a tour of the old Victorian town. We were in a daze of love, happiness, and good wishes, and we were husband and wife. The driver clucked his tongue and the Clydesdale began a slow ramble through the quaint, weatherworn town. We felt like royalty, the center of attention as strangers stopped to wave. And we waved back as if in a dream. I whispered to Bob, "Is this for real?" Little did I know how very real our life together would soon become.

While our carriage did the town tour, the AVM was readied for our reception. Tables and chairs were rearranged. A long buffet table decorated with flowers was laid with our offerings of smoked salmon rolled with dilled cream cheese, dolmas, fresh fruit, crisp green and potato salads. Others placed dishes they'd brought, and in the center of it all was our wedding cake – three tiers, one each of chocolate, carrot, and raspberry, swathed in French vanilla butter cream. We returned to the sound of popping champagne corks and the icy golden liquid tipped into tulip glasses.

Helen officially toasted us, telling everyone in her carefully chosen measured words what a good friend Bob had been to her and how she hoped we three would continue to be. She then took credit for having pushed us together when she could see what we couldn't. Our relationship was a point of pride for her.

Through all the well wishing, hugs, smiles, photos, and laughter both Bob and I were independently aware that Helen's fifteen-year-old daughter, Lisa, was quietly belting down the contents of unattended glasses. Helen was either oblivious or didn't care and we were too preoccupied to give it much thought.

***

It felt like we'd been on one continuous honeymoon from our romantic beginning nearly two years earlier, when Bob arrived on Filicudi. Hungry to explore together, we'd traveled to Hawaii, Mexico, and England. So after the wedding we decided to stay home. A honeymoon felt anticlimactic. Instead, we set about changing everything. Within two months we'd sold Bob's house and moved to the San Francisco Bay Area to share a home in the Oakland hills with Helen and Lisa.

After a disastrous year living with her father, Lisa wanted out, but she wanted to finish her last year in the high school she'd been attending. And Helen, a busy physician who traveled frequently administrating the programs she'd developed, needed help. We volunteered.

I'd never lived in such a house. It was modern and spacious, with high ceilings and big windows opening to a view of the forest surrounding us. From the kitchen, we could see a wedge of San Francisco between the hills. I arranged my painting studio in the dining area and set to work.

I planned not only to paint steadily, but also to promote myself as an artist. The art world was changing rapidly and required an artist to spend at least as much time in some form of publicity as in creating. I could paint up a storm, but the mere thought of selling myself turned my stomach into a burning knot.

Bob found a job in the window-covering business in Marin County, an hour's drive from home. He was no longer self-employed, as he'd been most of his adult life. "It's challenging to give so much energy to someone else's enterprise," he told me.

But two years of gallivanting about the world had depleted most of our savings. "I wouldn't give up an instant of our adventures,' said my husband. "Don't worry, love, this job is only a stepping stone."

So there we were, newlyweds in a new house, in a new town, when just three weeks into this arrangement we discovered that Lisa was addicted to drugs and alcohol – not one, but both.

The Mad Hatter ride began.

***

On her counselor's advice and with Helen's prodding, Lisa went to either Alcoholics or Narcotics Anonymous every day, often telling us later about the meetings. We wanted to see this as an endeavor to stay sober, but something didn't feel right. It was as if she was going through the motions to please her mother, who thought this was an easy problem to fix and didn't honestly believe her daughter was an addict. But Lisa confided to Bob and me, "These meetings might not be enough. I can say, 'Hello, my name is Lisa and I'm an addict,' but in my heart of hearts I don't really believe it. I honestly think I can use drugs recreationally and I'll be able to quit when I want to." She paused, gazing out the window for a minute. "The problem is, I think I want to be sober, but in reality I'd rather be high."

Lisa was bright and had an almost photographic memory, which made schoolwork a breeze. And she was fun to be with when she wasn't engaged in druggy behavior, which rendered her snippy, selfish, and manipulative. At these times, she often belittled us in front of her friends.

"Susan, Jeff and I need a ride to the Bart Station."

"I'm in the middle of a painting, Lisa. Can't Jeff take you? I thought he brought you home."

"He did. But now he's stoned and we want to go to a meeting. You don't want him driving, do you?" And then, in a stage whisper to Jeff, "My Mom pays for this house – Susan has to do it."

The heat of anger started to rise in me - for the lie, for the manipulation and for having my work interrupted again. I pushed it down and got my car keys.

We all wanted to believe this was a phase Lisa would grow out of, that this was peer pressure she would see through, but soon the situation reached critical mass and denial was no longer possible. "How did this happen?" became our mantra. But in the end, how it happened didn't matter. What did matter was whether Bob and I would stay and plunge down the rabbit hole with our two friends, or go, leaving Helen to handle the situation on her own.

As strong as the urge to flee was, we both felt we had to stay and finish our fourteen-month commitment. Bob had lived with these two women for four and a half years. He wasn't only a loyal friend; he loved them as family. Helen teared up when we told her. Lisa reverted to her childlike self and squealed with joy, flinging her arms around Bob's neck.

Early into the arrangement I'd written in my journal, *Truth, absolute Truth, is the most important thing in my life. To be one with That, I'll go wherever and do whatever is asked for. I am ready to clean out my mental cobwebs so I can feel truthfully.* To me, absolute truth is what is real in this very moment - not what we think about it, or how we judge it, but what is. For me, That is synonymous with God.

Staying with Lisa and Helen seemed a good way to jump into a cleansing fire and burn away all my outmoded thinking. Bob, too, was willing to break through boundaries and comfort zones. So when people told me how lucky Lisa was to have Bob and me, I felt we were the lucky ones to have this opportunity for growth in our lives. But that resolve was to be nearly blasted to bits in the months to come.

It was the most painful year of our lives together. The intensity was unrelenting as Bob and I confronted our conditioning, triggers, weaknesses and strengths, digging deeply into our psyches and exposing ever more issues while we tried to support Lisa and Helen.

Lisa was deeply attached to Bob. They'd lived together for four of Lisa's formative years when Helen and Bob were a couple. Helen was often out of town for work commitments, leaving them to strengthen their emotional bond and work out living together while she ran her business.

"Sometimes I felt like a glorified babysitter," Bob told me. "Lisa would be on the phone to her mother a thousand miles away, protesting because I'd set a limit on some activity. She wasn't used to someone saying, 'No'."

Bob set boundaries good-naturedly, but set them he did, and Lisa always knew where she stood with him. She loved him even more for that, and respected him. More than once Lisa sat on Bob's lap with her arms around his neck and told him, "I think of you more as my Dad than I do my real father."

Michele and Dawn, Bob's own daughters, had taken Lisa on as a little sister. There were family trips to Hawaii and Club Med in Mexico for diving and trips to the mountains for skiing. But after some years, the intimacy Helen and Bob shared became strained, leaving a residue that evolved into a best-buddy friendship. When Bob moved out, they talked on the phone almost daily, supporting each other through dark hours, but the candle of passion had burned the length of its wick.

***

The situation in the house grew tense with teenage boys climbing in and out of Lisa's bedroom window and Helen standing up for her from afar while we were the ones responsible for her day-to-day living. It was as though she was acting out to push the limits as far as she could. Bob saw what was happening. "It's obvious that she's desperate for Helen's attention, but no matter how outrageous her actions, it's never enough."

Bob felt powerless to help, and that powerlessness saddened him. He and I remained united in our feelings about what we were experiencing. We couldn't understand how Helen could still be in denial that her daughter was on a dangerous trajectory.

The unstable situation drove us to individual therapy, couples' therapy and family therapy for the four of us. Finally, when Helen couldn't deny any longer that her daughter was in deep trouble, she sent Lisa to live in a residential rehabilitation center. Lisa found comfort and safety being with other addicts and quickly built camaraderie and pride in being one with them.

Once a week we spent a full day of excruciating emotional pain listening to many of the teens in this unit reveal the sexual, physical, and/or emotional abuse woven into the fabric of their families. I spent most of these sessions silently crying, feeling my heart was shattering. Sometimes I wanted to run so I wouldn't have to hear any more tragic dramas like the story of the child whose mother burned him with an iron when he was 'bad' until he grew big enough to defend himself. The experienced therapists were trying to start the mending process within the families but the traumas ran so deep it seemed as challenging as climbing Mt. Everest blind.

Although my life had been easy compared to most of these kids, some of the milder stories echoed parts of my own childhood growing up with an alcoholic rage-aholic father. Memories broke loose that I thought were safely locked away, like the time he hit me so hard that my sister, Joan, was afraid I'd have detached retinas.

To this day I still have to force myself not to eat quickly, but to slow down and savor food. As a child, the dinner table wasn't safe. I didn't know from night to night if I would upset my Dad by talking about the 'wrong' subject, incurring his wrath. Most nights I finished as soon as I could and asked to be excused, running to the safety of my room. Even now I have an adrenaline rush when I hear anger expressed publically.

When I was fifteen my dad, already well lubricated, was driving me to a close friend's house for a party. Even though it was only a five-minute drive on dark quiet streets, I was afraid as he swerved the car towards our destination. I just wanted to get there. He was so out of it he didn't see the black dog in the road and ran right over it. The dog howled in pain. I was sobbing uncontrollably. As he lifted the dog into the car to take to a vet, it bit him. I was secretly glad.

When he dropped me at the party, I had to tell Dorene that we'd just run over her beloved pet. I didn't speak to my father for a week, mimicking my mother's way with anger. Inkie had to be put down.

In that year of intense inner work in California, I not only began to understand that my father's alcoholism had greatly affected me and that I'd been in denial about it, but thanks to an excellent therapist, I was able to accept my Dad, love him as he was, and understand he was never going to be equipped to be the father I wanted. He did the best he could. That was one of the greatest gifts of that year of being open and vulnerable so much of the time.

***

The first time I remember being that emotionally naked happened when I was sixteen and sitting at my favorite spot on a breezy Bolinas cliff top overlooking the crashing surf below. I often went there to think. On that particular day, a flock of pelicans were floating in the calm beyond the waves.

Suddenly, as though a signal had been given, one bird rose up, silently inviting the others to join it. Soon, they were all swirling through the air, circling, each on its own course until one dove straight down, wings flattened against its body and disappeared under the surface. Another dove, and another, then more than I could count, each pelican surfacing with a fish in its bill. The sky was a circus of acrobats rising up, circling, diving, rising up, circling, diving, and as I watched, time cracked, revealing a moment of infinite wonder. My heart burst with bliss, tears streamed down my face, and the landscape of my life changed forever.

Searching to understand this experience, I started meditating daily in my early twenties. Meditation brought a sense of equanimity to the chaos of life. But that emotional roller coaster year with Lisa and Helen pushed me off-center. I swung from euphoria one day to frightening anger the next, which left me in despair that I would never feel normal again. I so wanted to be compassionate and caring of Helen going through this Hell with her daughter, but instead I found all my buttons were not just pushed, but taped down in the 'on' position. Meditation didn't help.

When Bob and I first started living together, I continued my practice of twice-daily hour-long mediations that I'd done for years. I didn't talk about this unless he asked because I didn't expect him to embrace the practice, but eventually he started to question me and finally asked me to teach him to meditate. He took to it easily, so by the time we started living with Helen and Lisa, Bob was used to having that quiet time in his life. And he made sure he got it. Mellower than I to begin with, he didn't take things as personally as I did and rolled more easily with the waves of upheaval, waves that I resisted.

I also resisted Helen, a highly controlled woman. We were opposite in so many ways. I'm fire. She was ice. She was rational. I'm intuitive. It was a confusing and explosive cocktail of personalities. She was also the Queen of Double Messages.

When we hadn't seen her for a few days, we'd hug her and welcome her home. She'd sit at the table with us and ask, "What have you two been up to since I've been away? Tell all!"

We'd tell her of bike rides after work, discovering new parts of Berkeley, the painting I was working on, or new restaurants to try, but almost always her attention would stray to the mail or newspaper between us. She'd flip through it and stop to read an article, leaving us in mid-sentence. My teeth would clench as anger rose and I'd try to push it back.

Bob, our Mr. Mellow, or Plain Vanilla as he refered to

himself, took all this in, observing and monitoring. "Wouldn't a stroll along the marina be nice right now, Suz? I'll bet the sunset will be spectacular." He'd kiss me on the cheek, dissipating my anger, and we'd leave Helen to whatever distraction had taken her from us again.

In spite of Helen telling us from time to time that we meant a lot to her and she loved us, distrust started to build. This happened for me more quickly than for Bob, who was going through his own identity crisis trying to make a living anew in his mid-fifties. But he was still able to be our grounding wire, holding the swirl of emotions gently, with down-to-earth equanimity.

Bob couldn't always articulate what he felt, but he had radar for how I felt. He felt responsible for us being in the house even though it was a mutual decision, and he was protective, wanting to shelter me. When I'd have a meltdown, he worried that he'd gotten me in over my head. I, of course, protested, fearing he thought I was weak.

In the midst of the maelstrom, Bob and I went out for Sunday breakfast. Holding hands across the table waiting for our sunnyside-ups, crispy home fries, and fresh apple muffins, he looked deeply into my eyes, "I've always wanted to be a successful man. I used to think that meant money. But with you as my wife, I feel I am successful." There we sat with silly grins and tears pooling in our eyes.

One of the hardest aspects I was trying to master was accepting that anger is just an emotion, and it's the stifling of the rising heat that gives it so much power. I was desperately afraid that if I didn't control my anger, I'd be like my father. And yet everything I experienced was showing me that keeping a lid on the steaming pot wasn't working. I had to allow and observe the emotion, and in that awareness the anger would change. It took all the courage I could muster to change my relationship to anger, but in that change I occasionally found peace.

As I've travelled the spiral of life, I've encountered this situation again and again, each time a little wiser, but there has never been a definitive end to my struggle with this sticky emotion. Yet the lessons from our time with Lisa and Helen were an enormous help when Alzheimer's came into our lives fourteen years later and patience escaped my grasp again and again.

***

When Lisa graduated from high school in June, it felt as if Helen, Bob and I deserved diplomas as well. We four were forever changed, deeply connected in ways we could never have imagined. Although our friendship with Helen had teetered on the verge of ruin during this trial by fire, it was to endure until Helen lost a valiant fifteen-year battle with cancer twenty years later.

I reflect on how that torturous year affected us and I count the gifts it brought. It could have driven Bob and I apart, but instead it fused our relationship. It forced us to face our demons and our weaknesses and to pay tribute to our strengths. We'd seen the most vulnerable parts of one another, the ugly, deplorable components we hoped no one would ever notice, and we'd supported each other in accepting those segments and loving one another in spite of them. It wasn't easy, but our love helped us scale those high walls of challenge and rendered us more deeply in love than we thought possible.

Looking back, I see how that year prepared us for our next great adventure. Had we not moved into the house with Helen and Lisa, we could have easily kept running in the squirrel cage of work, going round and round to support a comfortable life, but never venturing off course to taste untried delicacies. But I'm a risk-taker and Bob was a willing partner. We joined hands and leaped into the unknown.

Chapter Six
Love At First Sight

Asia called
Beckoned me with crooked finger
And I came running, hesitant at first
Careening full bore at last
Master of duality
Compelling repelling
Beguiling mysterious ugly and decayed
She has me in a vice grip yelling for more
Head back eyes open
I take in her scents her sounds
Callousness rubbing my white skin raw
Rawness a portal to vast new vistas

With our commitment in Oakland finished, we were ready for new vistas, ready to hit the South East Asia backpacker trail. We crammed all our possessions into a storage unit and snapped the padlock into place, expecting we'd be back in a few months to make a new home in the States.

When we stepped out of the taxi into the evening carnival of Bangkok's Khao San Road, our first stop in Asia, the sensual assault ran away with us. The smell of frying chilis caught in our throats. The pervasive aroma of ginger and fish sauce near the street stalls drew us in to listen to crackling gas flames heating red-hot woks. The glittering lights, and scores of tattooed, pierced, or dreadlocked backpackers milling about captivated us. Hill Tribe women in brightly colored embroidered and beaded traditional costumes dazzled us with their handicrafts. "You buy this, Madam?" one of them asked, her hand reaching out to stroke the blonde fuzz on my arm.

Bangkok was hyper-alive and we were on fire. We dropped our bags at the first hotel with an available room, a room with a bed-length mirror hung low on the wall. Bob winked, wrapping his arms around me, "I hope this mirror isn't two way."

The room and the mirror would have to wait. We were anxious to return to the kaleidoscope outside. It was eleven p.m. and in spite of traveling for thirty hours we were eager to explore this Venice of the East. Shops, cafes and travel agencies lined both sides of the street, which was closed to vehicular traffic. German, English, Austrailian, French, Italian, Hebrew, Spanish, and Malay mixed with the sounds of the Thai language to form a symphony that delighted our ears. Asia was love at first sight.

***

At a breakfast street stand with a few small folding tables and plastic stools, we began our long-lived infatuation with *congee*, a thick rice porridge introduced by the Chinese. Ours had a raw egg, coriander leaf, shredded ginger, and what we think of as crullers, deep-fried bread dough, perfect for adding crunch to the soft soup. Each Thai diner flavored their bowl with fish sauce and pickled chilies from small glass jars set on the table. We were the only Westerners.

Fortified, we taxied to Chatuchak and made our virgin foray into the sprawling thirty-five acre, sense-assaulting, anything-you-could-possibly-want, mother-of-all weekend markets. We wove through throngs of people and goods, ogling, smelling and touching old and new Chinese porcelain, silks, Burmese gongs and tapestries, knives, amulets, herbs, dried fish, fresh fish, aquarium fish, pillows, quilts, Hill Tribe crafts, jewelry, birds, puppies, fighting-cocks, new clothes, used clothes, pineapples and papayas and watermelons, fried scorpions, and crunchy grasshoppers served with sweet chili sauce. Our heads were spinning and we'd just gotten started.

Enchanted, I longed to start bargaining, to fill up our bags with the finely-made, colorful crafts that were piled high in stall after stall. Instead, we stopped at a drinks stand to fortify ourselves against the sticky heat with Thai iced tea. It came in tall glasses poured over crushed ice, scented with vanilla and sweetened with condensed and evaporated milk.

"You know," I said to Bob as I slowly stirred my tea, "people at home would love these things. Those chunky silver necklaces we were looking at, the handwoven bags, those bamboo baskets you liked. I've never seen anything like them at home. What if we took some back to sell?"

Bob laughed and winked at me. 'Well, if nothing else we'd have fun shopping together."

For me, it wasn't entirely a new idea. On trips to England I'd bought hand-knitted designer sweaters and held home parties to sell them when I returned. Though I hadn't made a lot of money, it had been enough to cover travel costs. I looked at Bob, who was lost in thought, and wondered if he was taking me seriously. When we'd left Helen's, we'd agreed we needed to lighten our load materially as well as psychologically. But that was before we'd seen what Thailand had to offer.

"Other people do it," I said. "Why couldn't we?" I was lining up my arguments, about to remind Bob that if we wanted to go on traveling, we had to find a way to make it pay. But Bob was already ahead of me.

"We wouldn't need to own these pieces," he said thoughtfully. "We could have the fun of bargaining for them, and we might keep one or two, but you're right - I think we could easily sell what we bring back." He reached across the table and squeezed my hand. "And if something really speaks to us, we could keep it for a while and then sell it."

And so, on our first morning in Bangkok we clinked our sweating glasses in a toast to the birth of our new business. Over another round of tea we chose the name *Savoir Flair* and began to work out what we could afford for its fledgling inventory.

***

Sometimes the city's stifling heat rendered us grumpy even though we had frequent cold drink stops. Our different styles of crossing Bangkok's busy streets, where the pedestrian does not have right of way, set Bob on edge. Pedestrians had to scoot as quickly as possible and I'd lose my nerve midway while Bob was waiting, frustrated, on the other side. "Why can't you just trust me and go when I go?" he'd ask. But I found I couldn't. If my life was in danger, I had to be in control. This came up time and again throughout the Asia trip. We made a peace pact that he would work on patience and I'd work on trusting him more.

Bangkok's legendary Buddhist temples, called *wats*, are sanctuaries and a good place to cool one's irritation. The polar opposite of Bangkok's hot, chaotic exterior, they're quiet and serene, and they beckoned us in to sit in silence when the stimulus of the streets and the pollution reached overload. Inside, we were often gifted with the unexpected, like the day we encountered a flock of nuns chanting hypnotic refrains from the Buddha's dharma. Their cadence seemed to peel away the over-stimulation of the city, and like snakes shedding their skins, we felt born again into an inner world of quiet observation.

No matter whether it's a Thai wat, an Italian cathedral or a Hindu temple, places of worship hold a special ambience for me. Perhaps it's the centuries of worship, the sheer volume of people praying to a higher power, that imbues the space with sanctity. Whether or not I believe as the locals do isn't important. As I settle into the space, I sense something beyond beliefs, beyond them-and-us, beyond thought, a place of silence open to all who care to brush up against it.

Bob, however, soon became wat-weary and put a limit on how many we could visit in a day. He was like an active boy, wanting to explore and see and do. Our regular meditation was enough for him. I tried to tempt him with promises of treasures inside, but relationships need compromise, and so we eventually found a balance of shopping for Savoir Flair, exploring, savoring, and 'wating' before it was time to leave Bangkok.

***

The second-class air-con car seemed a good choice when we boarded the eastbound train. Neil Diamond on the sound system was a bit dated, but mellow, and he was one of Bob's favorite singers. We settled in with cold drinks and snacks. But once underway we were suddenly bombarded by C-grade horror films blasting throughout the car. Earplugs came in handy for the next four hours, keeping the decibels down to manageable levels and allowing us to read, but I'd glance up now and then to see decapitations, monsters, and enough oozing red to resupply an inner-city blood bank.

The train deposited us in the dusty eastern Thai town of Korat. We were there to visit the Khmer ruins at Phimai, part of the ancient Khmer empire centered at Angkor Wat in Cambodia. Phimai, built in the 12th century, was the birthplace of a succession of Angkor kings. We'd come to drink in the inspiration they'd left behind.

Entering Phimai, we crossed the Naga Bridge decorated with hooded serpents symbolizing the journey from the profane to the sacred. As we passed under laterite lintels and rubbed our hands along ancient columns, I thought: *It's just as I remember it*. I felt I knew the place. And I felt comfortable there.

Repeatedly, Asia would present me with the sensation of being more at home than ever before, rather than in some foreign, exotic land. I confessed to Bob, "My earliest childhood photos show a tow-headed blonde with almost Mongolian eyes. 'How did the Asian get in there?' became a family joke."

Bob laughed. "There's more to you than meets the eye. What did you say your name was?"

From the center of the main temple at Phimai, doorways radiated out in four directions, forming an equidistant cross. We sat alone in the transept, closing our eyes, feeling the earth and the heavens meet in our bodies. Another thought formed: *You're on a pilgrimage. Enjoy each step of the way.* Tears rolled down my cheeks, a familiar sign that I'd encountered something deeply true for me, a life changing event. And we would eventually see how life-changing this trip was, even though we couldn't fathom it just yet. We had to live it and grasp the outcome later.

We traveled to see more Khmer ruins, stationing ourselves in the small town of Buriram, where the hotel receptionist found us a driver without a speck of English. He took us down long, gravel roads, billowing dust in our wake, past water buffalo reflected in flooded rice paddies, through tiny hamlets and lush vegetation, finally depositing us at Phanom Rung. This vast ruin is perched on the rim of an extinct volcano with sweeping views of the valley below.

A pillar-lined path leads to stairs where more five-headed *nagas*, or water serpents, greeted us as we climbed. This Hindu shrine, once a monastery, is dedicated to Shiva, the God of Destruction. Carved on a lintel are his partners in the Hindu trinity: Vishnu, the Maintainer, and Brahma, the Creator. In Hinduism, creation, maintenance, and destruction go hand in hand, the cornerstones of life in this ever-changing universe.

Maung Tom, unlike Phimai and Phanom Rung, had not been restored. Even though it was nothing more than piles of posts and lintels and tumbled-down stones with faint hints of decoration

- the rubble of time passing – it had a peaceful atmosphere. I found all three of these temples inexplicably soul-nourishing.

Back in Buriram we wandered the night market purchasing fruits we'd never seen: red, spiky rambutans with juicy, translucent white flesh and mangosteens with thick, dark purple skins housing segments of indescribably delicious taste. Everywhere we looked, we were greeted by smiles. Sellers would reach out and touch us during a transaction. Bob suddenly got teary-eyed, feeling his heart break open amongst these people, especially the elderly. He said, "They've seen so much, worked so hard, and they go on and on. Even when distorted by disease and time, their faces are beautiful."

Our journey had become one of seeking a new way of being, a new way of living. We felt like open vessels ready to catch whatever rained over us, knowing we could filter out later what didn't fit. Yet questions of destiny dogged us, revisiting when we least expected them. We were gestating, brewing, and a bit impatient, wishing for a crystal ball to see the future. In the end we took a deep breath and surrendered, enjoying the passing scenes that each moment brought.

***

We reached Chiang Mai at seven a.m. after a rock and roll night down the train tracks. With hard bargaining we hired a three-wheeled tuk-tuk to take us to Lek House, a small inn with a large central garden where we'd breakfast, take respite from the afternoon heat, and sometimes dine.

We spent our evenings building the stock for Savoir Flair's cache at Chiang Mai's famed Night Bazaar. We found wall hangings, jewelry, clothing, shell belts, a monk's brass bowl that rang melodically when tapped with a smooth wooden peg, and our big splurge, a teak elephant chair that we shipped home, not realizing we'd never again have a home in the USA in which to put it.

We explored by day, venturing out to a Hmong village in the mountains. I felt like a voyeur looking at the rarely bathed population, the children with runny noses and tattered clothes, and a father of six, addicted to opium, unable to work. His wife had to do everything on her own and would eventually bury her husband when he'd smoked himself to oblivion, a common problem among the Hill Tribes. We bought well-crafted appliqué pillow covers made by the women, not even bargaining, holding back our emotions, and left feeling somber.

***

Custom's officials boarded the southbound overnight train from Bangkok, searching almost everyone's luggage. Drug smuggling is punishable by death in these Southeast Asian countries. The conductor had already collected our passports and turned them over to the immigration officials. We disembarked en mass and waited for our names to be called in this no-man's-land between borders. Rock music, piped out over loud speakers, competed with a woman's voice calling out our names. Bob, impatient and practical, started repeating each name in his booming voice for the crowd to hear. Once called, an official questioned us individually before a visa was glued and stamped, "Thomp thomp!" into or our passports.

Welcome to Malaysia.

Our first stop, Penang, was a weatherworn outpost from Britain's colonial days. It's legendary for its architecture and street food, both influenced by Indian, Chinese, and Malay culture and a fusion of the three.

While our days were spent exploring and on the lookout for Savoir Flair inventory, my nights were spent in another sort of journey. It felt like I went to the movies every time I closed my eyes.

I once read, "Dreams are letters from God and most people never open their mail." That line impressed me so much that I started writing my dreams down, trying to decipher their meanings, and studying the postage stamps for clues to their origins. I knew that no matter how far we travel, there's no getting away from ourselves, even when we attempt to go incognito by forming new identities along the way.

Between my dreams and waking awareness I was confronted again and again with my internal baggage. I had dreams that left me feeling so alone and abandoned that I wondered if it was this basic sense of separation and aloneness in our lives that causes our underlying pain and fear.

There I was on a discovery trip of a lifetime with my beloved, meeting interesting and inspiring people and this annoying disquiet showed up. At the same time I saw how much I needed alone time, which felt like a rare, precious gift.

Bob, on the other hand, was opening layer-by-layer to an even more delicate and sensitive core. He was so touched by the people he met, whether they were other travelers or locals, that he was wonderstruck. People commented on his infectious smile. They felt welcomed in his presence and accepted for who they were. He seemed like a wizened soul meeting up with old friends once again.

***

Buses can be a curious form of transportation in South East Asia. We never quite figured them out. You often board an empty bus waiting for it to fill. It helps to have reading material stuffed in your bag to dull the anticipation. Finally, after an excruciatingly long wait, the driver revs the engine and proceeds, and you relax, thinking, "Ah, we're finally underway," until you realize you've passed the same yellow house and flea-bitten dog three times.

The bus may spend an hour going up and down narrow dirt lanes, stopping to pick up passengers at their individual houses rather than at a communal bus stop where everyone gathers at an appointed time listed on an official schedule affixed to a post. If three passengers live on the same street, they may be close enough to wave to each other and even carry on a conversation, but still the bus stops at each of their homes. Sometimes there's no passenger, only goods placed on board to ride solo to their destination.

We'd been on buses careening down highways only to have brakes slammed on and a passenger picked up in what seemed like Doctor-Livingstone-I-presume jungle beyond the asphalt. A hundred meters further we'd stop again to pick up another and another. Before the bus could get out of first gear, the buzzer would ring for someone who wanted off. Our patience thinned.

And why? We were, after all, on holiday with no appointments to get to, no life or death situations to defuse. Instead, when we could reflect and laugh at the experience and ourselves, we saw what a helpful service was provided to the citizenry. It was like having a communal chauffeur, with the conductor or driver even helping women with their parcels. By the time the bus took off it would be packed to overflowing, with young men hanging out the door and holding on one-handed, noses in the air like cocker spaniels.

So off we went, stop-starting our way to our next Malaysian destination. The first two buses were easy rides. The third was filthy with trash cradling our bags. Someone had puked in the seat in front of us. I read while Bob dozed, his sleeping body slapping back and forth against me round the curves so that I had to hold on tight. To our right sat an elderly Chinese, chain-smoking her way to oblivion.

The long bus ride gave me time to contemplate my creeping discomfort. Something was brewing inside and I couldn't quite sort it out. I couldn't interpret the vivid images that were filling my nights with untranslatable but still compelling hieroglyphics, sometimes coloring my whole day with their mood. I seemed to flash between reality and dreams, sensing they were desperately trying to tell me something, as if two people separated by thick glass were trying to carry on an important conversation unable to read each other's lips. I prayed for a Rosetta stone.

We'd severed security strings, longing for a life outside the conventional box, and hoping to earn a living in unexplored territory. Was this prickling just me being ill at ease with these fledgling ideas, shedding the old skin and feeling raw and vulnerable with the not-yet-formed one?

I've always been a risk-taker, starting with the choice to live the life of an artist, which affords little security. I once scrawled in black permanent marker on the ceiling of my aging Ford van a quote from the movie *Flashdance* – "When you give up your dreams, you die."

Because I dare to dream and go full throttle to live those dreams, it appears to the outside observer that I'm brave, but inside, turmoil stirs up fear. I struggle with the *Who Am I?* question and I worry about how I'll eat. I have fantasies of being a bag lady, destitute beyond belief, but still something drives me to pursue my visions.

After days of scrutinizing this tumult, I realized that at its core the creative urge was pulsing, trying to surface. For seven weeks it had been overshadowed by travel. Now poetry was forming - a bit clumsily, but forming still. Wordplay banged around inside my mouth like sweet lumps of candy in a flavor I couldn't quite discern. It wanted out. Poems guided my pen across journal pages into impressions of our travels as well as the inner recesses I was exploring. (Some of those poems head chapters in this book.)

As much as traveling nourishes me, using my creativity sustains my core. And to give vent to this need, I crave time alone. Sweet memories of being on my own in Filicudi burst to the surface. Necessity was haunting me, but so was the fear I'd push Bob away if I took what I so fiercely wanted. I needed to find a balance.

***

Thailand had inspired our fledgling business. From there, we'd shipped our first cargoes home. Malaysia gave us cities and beaches to explore, and we met other travelers, most of them young, giving their adventurous spirits freedom before they started a 'real life' of career and family. Some had been traveling for a year or more, working their way around the world. They were our inspiration, the wire cutters of our old rusting fences, but though they nourished our ideas, in Malaysia we found almost nothing for Savoir Flair. It was time for something different.

Neat and tidy, efficient and expensive, Singapore was a vast contrast to Thailand and Malaysia. Our first impression of the island state was that we'd strayed into a high-rise architectural contest set in a well-manicured emerald jungle. No untidy green here: chartreuse, moss, olive, viridian, lime, and jade were all set out in an orderly fashion.

With a long list of errands, including air tickets to reroute and others to buy, we hoped upon hope there would be letters for us in Poste Restante at the GPO, a grand, gray edifice near the river's edge. We weren't disappointed. But the news in a letter from Bob's daughter, Michele, brought up disquieting issues.

She wrote, "Lisa is in residential treatment in a hardcore rehabilitation center in the Timbuktu of Montana. Her drug habit returned right after you left. Plus she started dealing cocaine. Helen literally kidnapped her and whisked her onto an airplane and off to a 'Tough Love' facility where she'll be for weeks. Helen has been trying to keep this from you."

I thought I'd neatly framed and hung the story of Helen and Lisa on the wall of my mind, but in Singapore it fell, the glass broken, and I had to deal with the emotional pieces scattered at my feet. "No matter where I go, here I am," came to bite me in the ass once again. Helen's secretiveness felt like distrust and I questioned the depth of our friendship.

Bob fell quiet when I read him the letter. His sadness grayed the room. He despaired for both Lisa's emotional health and for Helen, who he knew was disappointed and ashamed. He saw clearly, now that we were not mired in living together, how Helen craved our approval, while we, blind to that, craved hers.

We weren't sure what to do: write immediately to Helen to show our support or respect her desire to keep this from us. Bob suggested we give it a couple of days to sort itself out. He was sure the answer would show itself. And in the end he was right.

We wrote a joint letter – well, I did the writing because Bob really disliked the actual process of putting ink to paper, thanks to the traumas he'd suffered in grade school. We crafted the letter carefully, making sure it expressed as positively as possible our sympathy for the situation. He had to reign me in from any subtle barbs or blame I might have snuck in due to the hurt I felt from finding this out from Michele. Bob wasn't hurt, just sad.

***

The shopping centers in the Lion City felt like temples to the material, and we wondered if, hundreds of years from now, archeologists would unearth these monoliths and think they were religious centers. The Singaporeans, it seemed, shop as a benediction. Judging by the hordes swarming these sites, it was the main leisure activity.

Touts frequently accosted us selling copy watches, copy tee shirts and copy anything one could imagine with a famous brand name. They didn't try to flog the pieces as originals, but refered proudly to their wares as "Copy watch, sir?" Finally, the straw that broke the camel's back approached us.

Bob pulled me down behind a parked auto. The tout saw us but came round the car anyway. "Copy tee shirt, sir?" The devil took hold of us and we leapt up shouting in unison, "Copy watch?" pointing comically to our wrists. We fell into peals of laughter but the poor fellow didn't see the humor and backed off as if in the presence of the dangerous and unpredictable.

The shopping bug eventually bit us too and we found two Buddhist amulets from Cambodia for Savoir Flair. A Tibetan refugee selling prayer wheels, brightly colored mandala paintings, and turquoise and silver jewelry also caught our attention. I couldn't resist some of his pieces and bargained him down to a reasonable price, duly impressing Bob, who was no longer sure when I was bluffing. Bargaining had become a ritual, a rite of passage, a gentleman's duel. In Asia it's considered a success when both parties are content with the outcome, even though one or both may feign grave injury in the process.

We stayed in Singapore for a week, mostly indulging in its array of foods, and then we were ready for more adventurous traveling. We missed being where the day was unpredictable, inviting us time and time again to stay present because if we didn't, we'd surely fall in a hole in the sidewalk or bang our heads into a pipe jutting out of a wall. We also needed a culture that produced more fertile, ethnic items for Savoir Flair.

Chapter Seven
The Island of the Gods

Sitting at edge of lotus pond
All green with rose spikes pointing to heaven
I sketch peace and tranquility
Echoed by the temple beyond
Bali is everything I'd hoped for
Although not untarnished by foreign influence
Making it more real
More accessible
We fill our days walking and dreaming
Wishing to take home this simple life
From our small thatched cottage
In the rice paddies
With fireflies as dinner guests
And a frog ensemble singing us to sleep

After a quick trip to Yogyakarta, Java, where we meditated in Borobudur, the largest Buddhist structure on earth, and visited the vast Hindu complex of Prambanan, both built before the 10th century, we were antsy to get to our final destination. We landed with wings of anticipation on Bali in late September 1987.

Temples, temples everywhere, had our heads swiveling, with

architecture like nothing we'd ever seen – the Baroque gone Hindu. We craned to see out the *bemo* windows as the local minibus whisked us north to Ubud, the artistic center of Bali.

Right from the start, Bali assaulted our senses with scenes of sublime beauty shifting to the incomprehensible, to downright ugly piles of garbage. We came upon an altar in the center of the road with a woman in a batik sarong wafting incense towards it. Traffic buzzed by on both sides, but she focused on her prayer, oblivious to the whirlwind around her. A hairless fleabag of a dog waited for her to finish and turn away so he could snatch the bit of rice she'd left in the palm leaf basket. The Gods have to be quick in Bali to accept the essence of these offerings before they disappear.

Mount Agung, Bali's most sacred mountain, welcomed us in ten thousand feet of volcanic majesty. Flooded rice paddies in the foreground multiplied the image in their reflections, reminding us that it hadn't erupted since 1963, when over the course of two months, two thousand people perished. We hoped the volcano would control itself while we were on the island.

We pulled into Ubud and started the search for accommodation. With Bob's need for a comfortable bed and my need for aesthetics it was a challenge to find a room. I usually deferred and then grumbled. Finally we found a compromise with a view of golden rice and a bed Bob could sleep on peacefully.

Our eyes snapped open just after sunrise on our first morning. The view came with a sound track. It sounded like someone being murdered or working up to an orgasm. We scrambled out of bed to investigate, and saw a small, graceful woman with a blaring voice whooping and calling, flapping her arms, and working herself into a frenzy to scare away the small birds that came to indulge in the ripening rice. She had no mercy for us sleepers, but amazing stamina. She would come every morning and could keep this up for hours.

The next morning, my forty-first birthday, I awoke grumpy. After a night of strange dreams, including ropes emerging from floorboards trying to tie my feet down, I knew the gift I wanted most on this special day: time alone to create and draw.

Unfortunately, this came with the usual price – guilt. Bob was nothing but supportive of me and easily entertained himself, often meeting new and interesting people, so it was my own fear that was fueling my apprehension. I ended up shutting down to him for a few days and then missed the affection we usually shared. Shutting down seemed to give me the space to ask for the solitude I needed. It was a harbinger of how I'd adapt when Alzheimer's kidnapped our dream.

I finally took off with my pad and pencils and headed for the lotus pond in the center of town, where I drew for hours. I was in heaven until a renegade monkey, broken loose from her cage and dragging her chain behind her, came charging into the pond, shaking leaves and lotus seed pods at me. I ignored her. I wanted to draw. But she wanted my attention, and the more I ignored her, the more obnoxious she became. Finally, with a great splash, she dived into the pond, leaving my drawing and me dripping. Laughter welled up, smashing my seriousness. *What a great birthday gift!*

***

Bali was alive with colorful ceremonies and we were quickly entranced. But we didn't want to just skim the surface of the culture. We wanted to understand the rituals, which often take on a circus-like atmosphere when the public is invited.

"Sarong, madam? Cold drink, sir? Wood carving? Verrry cheap!" The hawkers put us off when we arrived at a cremation, expecting a solemn affair. But we soon realized that, in Bali, cremations are a festival of life.

Cremation is the final rite of passage, the last in a series of essential rites that give structure to Balinese life. The Balinese believe a soul will be born again into another body and it's their duty to help relatives and neighbours move into their next incarnation through very specific rituals evolved over centuries. There's a feeling of celebration because families feel joy and great relief when their responsibilities to the deceased are completed, leaving the spirit free to move on to a new rotation on the wheel of life.

Twelve corpses were being burned that day. Some had been in the ground for years waiting for this group ceremony, for it's often too expensive for an individual family to do alone. The remains, each one name-tagged and swathed in layers of white cotton, were arranged on one side of the road, waiting for their families to complete the offerings before the journey to the cremation ground could begin.

Sunlight glinted off gold and florescent colored paper adorning the tower that would carry the remains. Live chicks peeped from freshly woven palm leaf baskets suspended from the tower like ornaments. The tension built. Everyone was waiting for the sarcophagi, giant red and black bulls that often took months to complete, built of wood, bamboo, and coconut fiber, and covered in black or red velveteen, to be carried down the street.

A man with a bullhorn shouted instructions and the sarcophagi moved off as the wrapped bundles were placed in the tower. Then men and boys hefted the tower's palanquin onto their shoulders. With a great shout, rationality evaporated into pandemonium as the porters whooped and shrieked, running and stopping and turning, and running again as they spun the tower in various directions to confuse the spirits so they'd not remain attached to the remnants of their bodies or try to find their way back to their previous homes. We onlookers were running as well, either in hot pursuit, or to get out of the way of the tower running amok.

Finally, we arrived at the cremation ground, sweat running in rivulets down our backs and chests. The sarcophagi bulls were standing at attention, ready to welcome the deceased. Embellished with gold, red, yellow, and white accents, the black bulls wore mirror-studded necklaces and had fiercely painted eyes and menacing horns. Some had erect red penises, bringing snickers from the little boys.

The contents of the tower were redistributed to the families and carried over their heads, many hands touching them reverently as the whole entourage circled their sarcophagus three times. Then the bulls' backs were opened and relatives set the remains inside along with handwoven ikat and batik textiles, Chinese coins and other offerings. Priests chanted as they liberally sprinkled holy water over the whole works and friends and relatives moved around taking photos. At last, the sarcophogi were closed, gasoline was poured over the tower and bulls and, poof! With the flick of a match, weeks of preparation costing great sums went up in flames. For us, it was a commentary on how fleeting life is, how transitory and changeable.

We stayed for hours. At the end, the burning bulls were pushed over, the embers stirred, and a ruckus ensued as relatives rushed to gather the remaining bones and search for Chinese coins. The bones would be crushed into powder and carried to the sea, where another ceremony would be performed, the final stage of the journey for these last human vestiges.

***

Having been on the road for nearly three months, we longed for a house with a kitchen. We missed our own cooking. We told everyone we met what we were looking for. Finally a waiter suggested we contact Mr. Rasman up a long flight of stairs in an area called Campuan on the edge of town.

We couldn't believe our eyes when we saw a new thatched bungalow sitting by itself in the rice paddies. It had a kitchen, a sleeping loft, a bathroom and acres of rice paddies to gaze at from the veranda. It wasn't available until the following week, but we paid an advance and booked it for the remainder of our Bali stay, the last month of our Asian Odyssey.

While we waited for the bungalow, we planned a motorbike tour of Bali. But first Bob needed a local driver's license. Agung, the man whose bike we were going to rent, arrived at seven in the morning, and in typical Balinese fashion, gave Bob all the answers to the written test and had him practice driving for five minutes. Then off they went for the one hour trip to the police station in Denpasar, the capital and largest city on Bali. The driving test itself took very little time and involved Bob doing figure eights and maneuvers through pylons, but waiting for signatures, stamps, and the paper license took hours. I took the opportunity to spend the time drawing at the lotus pond.

***

We settled easily into Ubud life, making friends and often running into them and going for a bite to eat. Phillip and Jette, a couple we'd met in Malaysia, arrived in Ubud soon after us. Phillip was English, Jette Danish, and like us, they were obviously very much in love. There were other new friends too, like Paul, a fellow Californian who made a living by exporting handicrafts from Bali. He warned us about export quotas for clothing and suggested companies he trusted for shipping. He was open with his information and encouraging about our new enterprise.

Canadian Tamara, regaled us with stories of teaching English in Japan. "They'll pay eighty bucks an hour for lessons from native English speakers," she told us, getting our undivided attention. "I work for three months and then come back to Bali or travel until the money runs out. Then it's back to Japan to refill the coffers." We tucked this idea into the 'how to continue traveling' folder in our minds.

With this new sense of community, Ubud already felt like home, but it was time to strike out and see more of the island. We left our over-stuffed packs with Mr. Rasman and took off.

I'm not very comfortable on a motorcycle at the best of times. But having a tube bag strapped to the back of the bike and a daypack slung across my shoulders left me even more nervous. Bob patiently instructed me, "You have to let go and give way to the curves and the centrifugal movement of the bike." I knew he was an experienced, safe driver, but it pushed all my control and fear buttons and took great determination for me to loosen up, let go and let Bob.

We went northeast, crossing through Gianyar and Klungkung, both bustling cities with heavy traffic. In Indonesia, the biggest, most powerful vehicle usurps the right of way, so overloaded trucks and buses hog the road, struggling up inclines and careening down descents, and everyone else is expected to get out of their way. I was terrified. But once out in a more rural area, my legs relaxed their vice-like grip on Bob and I began to enjoy the ride.

We cruised into the seaside village of Candidasa, which looked like a boomtown with construction materials constricting the main road down to one lane. Accommodation and restaurants were going up as fast as bamboo grows, everyone wanting to cash in on the tourist influx. Sadly, there seemed to be no planning for the future and the town's coral reefs were being decimated for building material.

A room on the edge of town seduced us to stay a few days. It overlooked a lotus-filled freshwater lagoon separated from the sea by a thin spit of sand. We dropped our bags and walked the beach in search of fresh grilled tuna, a local specialty.

The next day, baggage free, we set off to explore the

surrounding area. Bob looked James-Dean-wild-and-sexy straddling the big bike and I fell in love all over again riding down tree-lined lanes with my thighs hugging him and my arms wrapped tightly around his waist. Now that I'd let go, I felt taken care of and protected. In his element, Bob was confident, relaxed, and oh-so-male. It felt like he and the bike were extensions of each other.

We ventured up to the Bali Aga village of Tenganan. The citizens there have an ancient pre-Hindu culture, resistant to change, although they have electricity and television. They're known island-wide for their unique ceremonies and for their double *ikat* weavings. These have both the weft and warp threads wrapped with ties and dyed in multicolored patterns so that, as the shuttle weaves the weft through the warp, the designs emerge from both directions. They command a high price that, sadly, was not in Savoir Flair's budget.

We explored the village, neat and trim and understated, peering into open doorways and chatting with the locals, and eventually found our way to a temple with a huge banyan tree standing sentinel over the back entrance.

"Let's go up this trail a bit," I suggested, and then every so often, "Come on, just a little further."

At first I had to encourage a reluctant Bob, but once a Taurus is underway, there's no stopping him. When the path narrowed and I thought about backtracking, it was Bob who said "Come on, keep going!"

We climbed on up, out of the jungle cool into an arid landscape with sparse trees and scruffy shrubs. The sun was blistering, but the crest of the hill beckoned us forward. Behind us, the mountain fell away to a canyon below, small and distant. The fresh blue of the sea leached out to the horizon.

"I know we'll see something fantastic at the top," said Bob, luring me onward in spite of my doubtful glares.

At the top of the last incline, Mt. Agung rose up right in our faces from a valley green with rice terraces, and the city of Amlapura nestled at its feet. Still showing traces of the 1963 reign of terror, this mountain demanded respect. Humbly, we spread our arms to better sense its power and felt like birds soaring over a vast panorama.

***

Candidasa turned out to be a good base for day trips. We buzzed down the road past Amlapura to the ruins of Ujung Water Palace, a vast complex built for the enjoyment of the last king of what is now the regency of Karangasem. Little was left after an earthquake in the seventies, but what remained, perched on a hill, would be a perfect element in one of my paintings. Crumbling columns and a sense of ruin were frequent themes in my watercolors, symbolizing transformation.

I got off the bike to take photos and before long, curious boys surrounded us, egging each other on to get closer and reaching out to touch our skin. When teenagers arrived to heckle us, we sped off down to the coast and along a black sand beach. Everywhere we drove, we were greeted with "Hello!" We felt like celebrities.

Driving north through spotless villages and vast sweeps of rice paddies, we arrived at Tirtagangga, another water complex and legacy of Karangasem's last king. A welcoming café overlooked fountains, swimming pools and ponds with carp so big they looked like they could have your arm for breakfast. Ever the suckers for atmosphere and a good cup of tea, we found a table to soak in the view.

"I feel such gratitude, for this gift of Bali, I said to Bob. "And for the magic of us." His eyes danced in agreement as he kissed my hand.

On the road through Rendang to Besakih Temple we were awestruck at every bend and every new vista opening in front of us. Rice terraces scaled the sides of mountains with a green so intense in sunlight and shadow that we shivered in wonder. We saw waterfalls, rushing rivers and grass huts perched on impossible inclines. As we bounced around hairpin curves, leaning into the centrifugal force, I felt free and two hundred per cent alive. I hugged James Dean tighter as we wound our way back to Candidasa through the luscious scenery, arriving at twilight.

***

It was a long ride back to Ubud and our little house in the rice paddies. We arrived just before sunset. After unpacking and settling in, we sat on the veranda in the dark. Frogs serenaded us and the firefly ballet was well underway. We watched in silence until we couldn't keep our eyes open any longer.

The next morning we lazed around under our mosquito net, so warm and cozy we didn't want to get up. Finally, I padded out to the veranda to write down a dream and soak up the morning quiet. Slow to wake fully, I don't like to talk much before that first cup of caffeine, but as soon as I got comfortable, our landlord appeared from around the corner, eager to chat. I sensed he'd been waiting to pounce. Personal space and privacy are foreign concepts in this communal society. I tried to explain that I wasn't yet awake enough for conversation, but the concept fell flat. I prayed this wouldn't become a morning tradition.

At daybreak the next day, several young boys were yelling and clamoring to keep the birds away from the rice surrounding our house. This was too much! I asked them to stop and they complied, but sat and watched us do our exercises on the veranda. As always, Asia was challenging our Western values and concepts. It would take time for us to learn that we couldn't impose them on an Eastern culture, but needed to adapt ourselves.

But despite the cultural clashes, beneath the surface a slow magic was taking root, a deepening sense that somehow we belonged here. It wasn't just the beauty of the landscapes or the sensual feast of the cultural rites. It went beyond the friendships we were forming and the relaxed patterns of our days. There was something here that spoke to us both at a deeper level, and for me more quietly than what I'd felt in Thailand. Both these experiences gave me a sense of coming home. It would be years before I traced its roots with certainty.

I grew up with three expertly carved hardwood busts standing guard over our family. They were perched on the top shelf of my mother's glass and cherry wood cabinet in the living room. These traditional teak carvings depicted a young woman with an intricate headdress and a handsome Asian youth wearing a head covering tied from a square of cloth. The third sculpture, of dense ebony, portrayed a weathered old man. They sat like guardians of my budding imagination, always there in the background, always encouraging visions of exploration. Draped across the hall wall was a Javanese batik with deep earthy shades of coppery red, indigo, and bronze punctuated by ivory whites and a cigarette burn, a legacy from one of my father's drunken nights. These pieces were in my blood – they'd always been there. I knew my father had bought them in the late 1930's in Singapore when he was a young merchant marine, living full-tilt boogie.

These four pieces spoke to my inner depths. As a child I fantasized that, disguised as a boy, I could travel anywhere and see everything. I could travel to the ends of the earth in my father's footsteps.

It wasn't until after Bob and I had been living in Bali for ten years that I inherited these sculptures. I suspected they were Balinese, but couldn't confirm it until I peeled back the green felt my mother had glued over their bases and read the incised inscription "*Toko Bali 1932*".

Until recently, the Balinese didn't sign their names to art works. The creative endeavor was universal, not personal, and so the inscription only meant 'Bali Shop'. Peeling back that felt was a revelation, a moment of synchronicity and déjà' vu. By then I knew these figures as real people. I saw them daily in the market or on the street, working the rice paddies or going to the temple.

The carvings felt like a mythical bridge, a conduit, a seed

planted deeply. They found their way to me at a tender age and left a trail like gingerbread crumbs that led me to Bali.

***

Goose bumps rose on my arms as I watched the *Pedanda*, or high priest, take his ceremonial files out of their protective covering, chant mantras over them and over one of eight initiates lying on a bed covered with golden ikat cloth. The family waited pensively for the Tooth-Filing ceremony to begin, tenderly touching the initiate's feet in moral support when he put his head back, opened his mouth and the Pedanda inserted a block of wood to keep his mouth open. The arteries in the young man's neck betrayed his lack of composure as his heart beat furiously in anticipation of this rite of passage into adulthood.

The filing began. Each rasp sent a grimace onto the initiate's face. The edges of his front teeth were filed, the points of the canines softened, and the surface of the front teeth given a good working over. The Pedanda used finer and finer files to smooth out the work. Finally, he held up a mirror so the new adult could admire his reshaped teeth, now devoid of animal connotations. Fortunately, in these modern times, the filing is kept at a minimum so the enamel isn't destroyed.

The seven others waiting their turn had already been anointed, blessed, and sprinkled with holy water. They wore apprehension on their faces as the tension built.

We'd been invited to this private affair by Wayan, who worked at our first accommodation. He'd befriended us and the friendship continued even after we moved to Rasman's house.

The finale of the day was a banquet of special ceremonial

dishes, including *babi guling*, the famous roast pig, and *lawar*, a mix of vegetables, shaved coconut, and pig's blood. There were platters of fried noodles, mixed vegetables, chicken sate with peanut sauce, and baskets of white and yellow rice. Dessert was a slice of perfectly ripe watermelon. Our heathen teeth were perfectly happy munching food just the way they were.

***

Our breath splintered into gasps when we opened the door the next morning to a new and spellbinding view. The clouds that had huddled on the horizon since we'd moved here had cleared, revealing five mountain peaks jutting up into an impossibly blue sky. It felt surreal that a landscape so humongous, so spectacular, could be hidden, and then to awaken to it sitting on our doorstep. The island was revealing her secrets in layers, and as each layer peeled back, we wanted more.

Buoyed by this morning surprise, we motored into town to check our mail, but left disheartened. There was not a single letter. Even though we were living our chosen life and making new friends as we went, we missed family and friends at home. Contact with our loved ones kept us in the bigger picture and kept us grounded, lest our dreams carry us off. It felt as if we were straddling a river, one foot planted on each shore.

Just around the corner was Kokokan Crafts, where Ben, the American inspiration behind its clothing designs, cheered us up with his stories of expat living in various countries. This was the start of a long-running friendship with a man who'd have considerable influence on our life in the coming years. He both intrigued and inspired us with his travel tales, urging us on to live our dreams as he had his.

Ben produced colorful jackets with wide, dramatic sleeves banded in stuffed black satin, perfect for Savoir Flair. The body of the jacket was made from local hand-woven rainbow-colored ikat, called *pelangi*. We chose a half dozen to take back and a few dresses we were sure we could sell.

After business, the urge to create drew me back to the lotus pond once again. I couldn't get my fill of these strong but delicate flowers, which Buddhists believe symbolize purity as they rise through and above the mud of life to their full potential and then wither and die, symbolizing that everything in life changes.

While we'd been traveling around the island, the pink blossoms had grown so tall that they towered over me when I sat in the grass beside the pond to sketch. This gave a unique perspective with the light coming through the translucent petals and shadows playing on the green. I sketched for hours.

The monkey, broken loose again, came dragging her chain and sat by me. In her wake, four small boys silently glided in and sat so close we were touching. They watched me draw with such respect it felt like a sacred event, quietly discussing what I was doing until their attention span pulled them away to other adventures.

A flash of inspiration suggested I make Phillip a book of poetry and drawings for his upcoming birthday. I began immediately, using many of my lotus sketches as background for the poems. I vacillated between feeling blissful when the delicious momentum bathed me in creative juices, often keeping me awake at night, to feeling like a fool to think anyone would want to read my poetry or look at what I feared was mediocre art. Still, I pushed on with the project. Doubt has dogged me my whole creative life, but it's rarely stopped me.

It was after one of those sleepless nights that we dressed before dawn for a trek down to Denpasar to make phone calls to the States. Ubud wasn't set up for international calls, and with a fifteen-hour time difference between California and Bali, we needed to get to the telecommunications office early. In typical Indonesian fashion, the phone office had moved and street signs were few and far between, making the trip feel like a treasure hunt. Undeterred, we alternated betweeen searching and asking directions, gradually zeroing in on the new location until Bingo! We spotted it.

Even at this hour of the morning the office was packed and we were glad we'd brought books to while away the wait. Once squeezed into a booth, receiver in hand, we shouted to be heard above the static, entertaining the entire office with our conversation. Since there were three booths, there were three simultaneously bellowed conversations. This was chaotic Asia at its best. It brought back sweet memories of Filicudi phone calls and our budding new love.

It was only 7:45 a.m. when we finished our calls and we were famished. After an opulent English breakfast of eggs, bacon, toast, grilled tomatoes and mushrooms and cups of Balinese coffee with sweet condensed milk, we headed for Kuta Beach. I watched our bags while Bob bodysurfed. I envied his comfort in the sea and the ease with which he handled the big waves.

Although he tried to explain the logic of the waves to me, I didn't have his natural sea sense. My stomach knotted when he said, "If you're ever caught in a rip tide, don't fight it. Just let yourself be carried out and then swim parallel to the shore until you find a safe place to get out."

"Ya, sure," I thought, vowing to be happy walking the beach or sitting on the sand. Every month, at least one foreigner on Bali is sent home in a body bag from not having listened to Bob's advice.

Back in Denpasar, we had a repeat performance at the telephone office, this time trying in vain to reach Bob's daughter, Michele, who we planned to visit in Hawaii on our way back to California. There was no answer. But since we were already in the city, Bob introduced me to Arts of Asia, a shop specializing in ethnographic pieces and weavings from around the archipelago that he'd found on a solo trip.

We met Verra Darwiko and his wife Irawati, the 40-year-old owners of this museum-like shop. Irawati was a quiet but shrewd business woman while Verra was a natural teacher and storyteller. He mesmerized us with his adventures of sailing the Eastern Indonesian islands and finding religious aritfacts and antiques no longer valued by the islanders. There was a beaded fabric tobacco pouch from Timor that caught our eyes, a gourd decorated with shells and a rainbow of beads, and a beaded horsehair bag. Beads, a very important commodity throughout the region, were used as bride price and in burials, as well as for decoration. Many of those in Arts of Asia were over a thousand years old. Little did we know then that those beads, and many others, would eventually string our lives together with our dreams.

The next morning I woke up annoyed at nothing in particular and wanting some alone time, but Bob decided to clean house. He derived great satisfaction out of cleaning but he wanted my help and I was not in the mood. Instead, I went for a long walk in the rice paddies to walk off my bad temper, finally ambling into town and the lotus pond for another drawing session before gathering treats, including all the flowers I could pilfer along the way, as a peace offering.

***

Splat! I was on the veranda working on Phillip's birthday present when a pair of wet shorts came flying out of the bathroom and landed by my feet. I tried to ignore them but soon, splat, splat, splat, a succession of wet laundry was jettisoned out of the bathroom, splattering me with water. Finally, I heard Bob taking a shower and called in, "Aren't you going to hang up the laundry?"

"I thought my assistant would do that," he said, trying to get a rise out of me.

I took the bait and exploded, "You're taking me for granted! I do the cooking!"

Traveling for three months in close quarters was taking a toll on us. A distance had been growing, and romance was cringing in the closet. I prayed this was only temporary.

I knew I was responsible for a lot of the distance with my need for alone time and guilt over taking it. I felt shut down and self-protective, as if I was holding a part of myself back from Bob, and although I didn't like it, I felt helpless to stop it. I feared my irritability would impact our relationship when he responded in kind. We needed to talk, but both of us were avoiding the subject, hoping it would go away. The splatting laundry soaked off the impasse. When he emerged from the shower, we made up, wrung and hung together, and talked about what was bothering us.

"I'm feeling pretty insecure about how we'll make a living when we go back," said Bob as he pinned a pair of shorts on the line. "Plus, I feel dependent on you."

Wringing out a tee shirt, I was considering what to say when he turned towards me. "I'm so afraid of losing you. But at the same time, you're getting on my nerves. You seem to need to vocalize everything to anyone who'll listen. I want some things left private!"

I stayed quiet and listened for a change, taking in what he was feeling and trying not to be reactive.

"And it feels like it has to be your way or the highway. Maybe we need more time apart. I don't want to burn out our relationship. When it's good, it's so very good." My throat constricted at the thought that I was driving him away.

Bob, usually Mr. Mellow, tended to let things roll off, so I respected that this wasn't easy for him to say, especially since he belonged to a generation which found it hard to talk about emotions.

"I love you," was all I could croak out.

Work and earning a living were a large part of Bob's identity.

He hadn't suspected before we left that insecurity would surface. Instead, he'd imagined himself to be a free spirit discovering the world. Savoir Flair had grown into a way he could rationalize our travels and feel useful, but he'd been without a job for three and a half months and we had only another three weeks to go with no set job prospects for our return.

This 'work insecurity' still shadows Bob, even in the depths of Alzheimer's. He obsesses about making a living and has conversations about imaginary clients. If he feels pestered, he'll shout, "I need to work, leave me alone!"

***

The next day I couldn't wait to get to the lotus pond to do the last drawing for Phillip's book. I was going overboard, trying to make it the best it could be, seeing every little nuance in a critical light. *Is he really going to like these drawings? Are they amateurish? And what about my poetry?*

I'd been grappling with my identity as an artist. Was I attached to the label because it felt exotic? Was I wearing it as a disguise so no one would see the real me? Sometimes I felt like a fraud.

Help with these questions breezed into a cafe one afternoon in the form of Bonnie, a middle-aged Irishwoman who'd attracted my attention around town with her bohemian dress and long auburn hair. Bonnie wrote, painted, and exported Balinese paintings. I told her what I was facing.

"Doubt is part of the creative process and always has been," she told me. "Every artist worth their salt grapples with it, and those that don't are lying." But the question of authenticity was to haunt me from time to time for years to come until I finally got a grip on fear itself.

The day of Phillip's birthday, the electricity went off. We dressed by candlelight and made our way to Café Wayan, where he'd ordered *Rijsttafel*, a holdover from the Dutch colonial era. It's a celebration of dishes that can range from six to twenty, including the mainstay, rice, and usually includes Bali's famous smoked duck. We indulged ourselves to happy capacity and then Phillip unwrapped my gift.

A wide smile spread across his face. "I can't believe you made this for me!"

We all sat quietly as he read most of the poems out loud. I sat there wondering *Who wrote these?* Hearing them read by someone else, relief washed over me as I realized they came through me, not from me. *I'm not a fool, at least not this time,* I told myself.

***

With only six days left of our Asia sojourn, we went into high gear buying inventory for our fledging business. We explored Celuk, the silver and goldsmithing village not far from Ubud, going in and out of shop after shop, purchasing sterling silver earrings and pendants, some brushed with gold, to add to our growing collection. Granulation, a time-consuming technique where tiny balls of silver or gold are soldered into place to form an intricate design, is a signature of Balinese jewelry. It adorned most of the pieces we bought.

Back at Arts of Asia, we spent an afternoon with Verra and Irawati. Verra enthralled us with more tales of sailing the outer

Indonesian islands, picking up handicrafts and ethnographic pieces along the way, and stunned us with his collection of sacred gold pieces. One rectangular piece of gold from Tanimbar, about three inches long, was carved into a primitive man seated on a mat. Another was in the form of the Hindu Shiva. We felt honored that Verra was willing to let us handle these rare objects, which we did with reverence.

With the power out, as it frequently was in Bali, we did our buying by candlelight. We chose, among other things, a rattan baby carrier from Borneo completely encrusted with beads and shells worn backpack style with baby inside, so the mother's hands were free for work. Imbued with character and spirit, this one was about forty years old.

I imagined the three sculptures I grew up with flashing us the high five sign. "Even if we fail, we'll have fabulous objects to remind us of this trip," I breathed into Bob's ear as we leaned into a curve on the return home.

We spent our last day in Ubud picking up orders and tying up loose ends. Gathering a mask in one village, we sipped sugary tea with the carver's family, enjoying a last helping of Bali's sweetness. At Kokokan Crafts, the last of the jackets we'd ordered was ready. We made the rounds to say good-bye to friends.

With Ubud's rainy season full on, Jette and Phillip moved to Kuta, Bali's most famous surfing beach, before returning to Copenhagen and real life. We followed, craving the sun, needing to dry out, and hoping to see them one last time. We knew we'd miss this pair of free spirits who inspired us with the depth of their commitment to love and to each other.

Instead of a downpour on the morning of our departure, we were greeted with soft white clouds breaking up the sky's blue. The paddy surrounding our house was filled with women harvesting rice. They cackled and chatted the entire time, often heckling each other and raising a roar of laughter. Their cooperation laid the paddy bare in no time. Enchanted with their work ethic, I ran through a roll of film. Then reluctantly we boarded the *bemo* that would take us to Kuta, our hearts heavy at leaving this town we'd come to think of as home.

Sunday, the day of reckoning, came calling early. We slipped out to walk the wide, white sand beach, appreciating what Bali had given us and grateful for the people who'd graced us along the way. We had no doubt we'd be back.

In the fifteen-hours to Honolulu we got little sleep, but settled back into our seats, holding hands in a cloud of contentment, and replayed highlights from our last four months.

"That first night in Bangkok, how starstruck we were!"

"And how green taking that room with the mirror at bed height!"

"Remember the tea shop at Chatuchak?" We squeezed each other's hands. And the hairs stood up on my arms when Bob reminded me of the déjà vu experience at the Khmer ruins.

But of all the places we'd visited, it was Bali that had stolen our hearts. We were returning to the States altered. Perhaps the contrast was greater for Bob, who had never traveled extensively before and had never experienced spontaneity as we had in recent months. He'd opened to a whole new way of being, with new possibilities of earning a living. His natural openness thrived in this lifestyle. I was already a risk taker and now I had company.

Michele, Bob's oldest daughter, greeted us at the Maui airport in a flurry of hugs and kisses just a few days before Thanksgiving. The holiday was an apt ritual for us to acknowledge the gratitude we felt, especially as verification that we were on the right path manifested when we sold nearly a thousand dollars of goods before even hitting the mainland. We were on our way.

Chapter Eight
Reality Check

Blessed is the influence
Of one true loving human soul
On another

- George Elliot

A huge grin stretches across Bob's face when I walk through the gate after my respite trip to Italy. The newly arrived luggage clues him in that I've been away. "I am so happy you're back!" he beams as he wraps me in a hug. "It's great to be together again!" For five weeks the boys have been telling him, "Susan's in Bangkok on a visa run and will be back in two days." He never questions this.

He's so sweet and affectionate that I temporarily forget he has dementia, reacting as though this is the pre-Alzheimer's man. But once the suitcases are empty and stored, he forgets I was ever away. The grin and affection are replaced by repeated questioning.

"What's for dinner?"

My stomach tightens as I'm tossed back into reality.

My return coincides with *Galungan*, a three-day island-wide

Balinese holiday. Not only are we without business and house staff, but I'm also on full-time Bob duty during the day, with Nano or Ketut, Bob's carers, only sleeping in the house at night. I've been jettisoned from free spirit to caregiver while still immersed in the fog of jet lag. Everything seems exponentially more difficult.

My newly built sleeping cabin leaks and I wake with a daily backache from the borrowed bed, making patience difficult. After only a few days, that old displaced feeling resurfaces. I feel like a visitor in my own home, with no place to go for comfort, no place to relax and unwind.

We do everything we can to keep Bob's anxiety as diminished as possible, but lately he's more agitated in the evenings and insists on the doors and windows being shut. This is contrary to life in the tropics, where almost everyone lives outside and leaves their houses open for air. I try to reason with him, try to get him to compromise and leave one window open, but after a minute or two he gets up and closes it again. Our house feels like a sauna and I can't bear to stay inside for long. Bob and his caregiver sit on the couch sweating as they watch animal programs on TV. I try not to cry.

Even the veranda is off limits as an evening sanctuary. We used to curl up there and read, or rehash the day's activities. Now Bob insists the veranda and garden lights be switched off, so as soon as the Galungan holiday is over, I start escaping nearly every evening with friends, leaving Bob with his caregiver. It begins to feel like I've never been away, never had respite.

The nights are particularly challenging. Bob frequently

gets up anywhere between one and three a.m. and goes to the kitchen in search of food. He's probably harking back to having midnight snacks with his father when his dad would return from swing shift at the shipyards during World War II.

One night he wakes Ketut. "Where's my wife?"

"She'll be home tomorrow morning. She's still in Bangkok."

Bob gets dressed, puts on a jacket and roams the yard, waking me in the cabin from desperately needed sleep. Finally, he wanders up to the car park and sits on the ground to pet the dogs.

Ketut follows. "Bob, there's ice cream for you in the kitchen!" Bob's sweet tooth lures him back to the house, the ice cream forgotten by the time he reaches it.

When these late night wanderings escalate, I'm urged to give Bob sleeping pills, but I want to avoid this because it increases the chances of incontinence. I realise yet again what a blessing it is to have caregivers who are willing to follow Bob around and protect him wherever he wanders. I don't know how I could do this without them.

***

Our bathroom feels like a public urinal. Bob can't seem to hit the toilet, liberally sprinkling the rim and the floor. The smell and yellow drips of urine begin to annoy me even though we scrub it daily. One afternoon I find him wandering the house with a towel around his waist, looking glum.

"What's wrong, honey?"

"I peed my pants," he says, disheartened. "I didn't even know I had to pee. It just came out."

I get up and put my arms around him. "Poor baby," is all I can muster. My heart aches for him.

Later that day he and Nano come home from the gym. As he enters the house, Bob says, "I used to live here. I remember this place!"

"Bob, you do live here. This is our house."

Perplexed, he asks, "How long have I been away?"

"About an hour."

I can't imagine how disconcerting and frightening it must be to feel lost and unsure of almost everything, especially oneself.

Sitting at lunch a few days later he repeatedly asks, "Do you have someone who trims your trees?" followed by, "Your trees sure drop a lot of leaves! We don't have so many trees at our house."

My curiosity and the repetition finally get the better of me. "Which house is that?"

He looks perplexed. "You've never been to our house?"

"Who do you live with?" I ask cautiously.

He's silent, and then looks me in the eyes. "I don't know."

"Who do you think I am?"

"Susan!" he answers sharply, as though I'm an idiot.

"And who am I married to?"

Bob takes time to think, then answers tentatively, "Is it Bill?"

Bill is married to Bob's ex-wife, Clare. Bob looks at me wide-eyed when I tell him I'm his wife of twenty-six years.

I ask, "Where do you think you are?"

"In Bali?" he says, unsure of himself.

"Where do you live?"

"In Bali!" he answers more confidently.

I take his hand. "Bob, can you tell me what's happening when I ask these questions?"

"My mind's just blank. There's nothing there." He looks beseechingly into my eyes.

"I'm really sorry, honey, but you have Alzheimer's."

I want to understand what's happening, how this disease works from the inside. It helps me feel more compassionate to have his personal interpretation rather than just what I've read in books. Usually, I try not to talk about the disease in front of him, try not to use the 'A' word, but occasionally I can't find replacements.

He looks confused. "How many children do I have? Where are they?"

When I say he has two daughters, Michele and Dawn, that seems familiar, but he has no idea where they live. He doesn't ask if they have children.

***

Besides the smell of urine, Bob's body odor has become acrid, but he's not aware of it. He long ago lost his sense of smell, a loss that's often a precursor to Mild Cognitive Impairment, the disease that he was possibly thought to have when we had him tested for dementia in 2002. At that time we didn't know that a significant percent of people with MCI go on to develop Alzheimer's. Where he used to be fastidious, sometimes taking three showers a day in these hot and humid tropics, he's now slowly becoming resistant to taking showers at all. Getting him in the shower is becoming a power struggle and I know I'm not handling it well.

"Honey you really need to take a shower." He takes forty-five minutes showing me choices of clothing to put on while I work at the computer. I say fine to anything, just wanting him to take the damned shower. But his 'clothes choosing button' is stuck in the on position and so he repeats and repeats this activity until I'm ready to scream. I can't concentrate on my work and do the shower dance at the same time!

Finally, I'm livid, "I won't eat breakfast with you unless you take a shower now!" I'm exhausted before we've even had our morning coffee, and though he's finally in the shower, I feel awful.

People with Alzheimer's can't remember facts, but they do remember emotions. I feel like a failure for having lost my temper once again and leaving my sweet man feeling he's in the doghouse for reasons he doesn't understand.

I'm also losing patience with my cabin. After only three months it's clear the foundation supports aren't strong enough, and now termites have come in droves, leaving mud trails marching up the walls. I try hard not to be depressed, but again the displaced feeling keeps hanging around. The house is clearly

Bob's territory. I need this small room to be my sanctuary, but instead it's my nemesis. It isn't safe to leave my laptop there for evening work because of the leaks and I can't work in the house because of the television and the heat.

And now, splat, splat, splat, rain is leaking through the roof and onto the bed. I wake up one morning to drips on my face and slither out of the way. Tears well up and add to my already wet pillow. I call the exterminator for the termites and the builder to have the roof removed and repaired for the third time.

I try to keep my focus on our business and remind myself that this is only temporary. Eventually, the cabin will be watertight and I'll have my oasis. In the meantime, I sleep at friends' houses for a week while repairs and fumigation go on. I long for a space to call my own. I long for a week of uninterrupted sleep. I long for normalcy. "I feel crazier than bat shit," I tell my friend Cat as I struggle to focus on what needs to be done.

Once the cabin repairs are finished, Bob continues to get up before sunrise, sometimes going to the workshop, which is right outside my cabin. Any noise he makes wakes me. Occasionally, he comes and knocks on my window, wanting to know if I'm there. I built the cabin as a remedy for sleep deprivation, but I'm still not getting the hours I need. I'm impatient with everyone, my staff included, and then I get impatient with myself for being impatient.

My wall of self-protection erects itself in an involuntary attempt to find some emotional space, but it gives me no comfort and shuts Bob out. Even though I know it hurts him, I feel powerless to stop it.

This happens for various reasons: answering the same question one too many times, having my focus pulled away too often, being stared at, or suddenly just not having any more to give. I watch the process, trying to understand it. I reach a point where it's all too much, something gets triggered and 'shut down' chemicals course through my body. I can see out, but I can't feel out. I'm trapped until the chemicals start to subside and I can warm up to Bob and be affectionate again.

Over the years I've had to adapt to keep Bob as happy and anxiety-free as possible. It's a one-way street. He can't give back because Alzheimer's has robbed him of that ability. He doesn't even have an inkling about the concept any more.

One night I ask him to give me a foot massage, hoping for a little comfort. He does his best, but he's robot-like, just going through the motions. In the end it becomes irritating to be touched so superficially, triggering more grief. I finally understand he can't help this. I won't ask again.

***

Ubud's been having rolling blackouts due to major electrical problems island-wide. I'm working in the kitchen by candlelight one night, with Bob standing off to the side staring at me as he watches me cook. He's bored and wants to be with me, but it's driving me mad.

"Bob, why don't you set the table?"

He seems happy to help, but I soon notice he's searching for the placemats. "Look in the top right hand drawer of the sideboard," I tell him.

With that done, he's looking for the cutlery. "Honey, the

forks and knives are on top of the small fridge." Without my constant guidance, he goes back to staring.

The shutdown starts. I know it's cruel, but I can't keep it from happening. I know he feels badly and feels he's done something wrong, but my rational mind is taken by quicksand.

In an email, my sister suggests a solution: "Turn on the TV." It works. Bob is engaged and I'm free to cook undistracted. Why couldn't I find this simple answer on my own?

Yet these hard times are sprinkled with humor and connections that keep me going. We usually have lunch together, and sometimes the conversations get me giggling, especially if I'm relaxed and able to go along with wherever Bob is in the moment.

Bob asks, "So how's your day going?"

"Just fine. How about yours?"

"I've been really busy."

"What'd you do?"

Bob forks a bit of salad. "Oh, I've been all around town. There's an auction I went to see."

"What're they auctioning?"

"It happens at the end of the day with all the stuff they didn't sell. Susan has stuff there."

"What does she have?"

"You know, the things she sells. Do you remember how much we made there last year?"

I grab a number from the air, quickly changing gears that I'm no longer referred to in third person, "About five thousand."

"I don't remember, but I thought it was more."

"I don't remember either."

Bob stares at his plate, "I guess I shouldn't be eating all this food."

"Why not?"

"I won't be able to sell it. I'd make more if I hadn't eaten it."

"But you're almost done, so you might as well finish it."

"Well, I should have put some garnish on it for when they come."

"It's almost done. Go ahead and finish it."

"When they come, I'll unzip my pants."

"Yes, and either scare them away or give them a good laugh!"

"I'll just hang it out when they pass by."

I have to laugh and wonder what on earth he's thinking. It's amazing how the mind works or doesn't work. And who does he think I am when he refers to Susan in the third person?

***

I don't usually throw money into my purse. I'm careful to always put it in my wallet and then put the wallet in my bag. But I was in a hurry today and tossed the bills into the open bag. This evening I find the money is missing. In its place are a copy of Bob's passport, a set of earphones he pilfered on our last flight together, and a pair of his dirty underwear. I chuckle over this for months.

When humor is there, or we have connection, I feel closer to him. There's a faint echo of how we used to be that brings up the old in-love feelings , a warmth that radiates out to him. I'll always love my gallant White Knight, but those old 'in love' feelings have drifted to the background and I miss them.

Occasionally, Bob makes sexual overtures, but he usually forgets what he's doing and so I carry on his advance. This has been our pattern for the last three years. But I find it increasingly difficult to feel sexual desire for a man I must care for and who's dependent on me like a child on his mother. Sometimes the body just demands, "It's time!" I've been home for a month and that time comes.

Lovemaking has become less and less successful in the last year. Viagra is not doing the trick, and since Bob has lost most of the feeling for 'the other', our old style of wanting to pleasure each other because we care so deeply, of really making love, has evaporated. Still, my body is ready and it seems his is too.

It's a warm, tropical night. We turn out the lights on the veranda and light a few candles. I take the lead since he loses focus easily, but it soon becomes clear he's confused and not sure what to do. He's forgotten what I like, and worse, what I don't like, and it seems he wants to do what turns me off. This is completely contrary to how he used to be. He was always more interested in giving pleasure than taking it, but now there's not a trace of this. I forget about myself and try to give him a good time, but his interest wanes and the whole fiasco turns out to be so emotionally taxing that I realize we can't do this anymore. I'm not ready to be celibate, but it's just too painful to try this again. I feel I'm taking advantage of him, taking advantage of someone no longer able to make his own decisions.

I so miss the deep connection that can only come with an intimate partner. I have plenty of connections with friends, and deep ones at that, but with an intimate partner something else happens. It's like having a third being between the two of you, greater than the sum of your parts. It's nurturing and helps get you through the hard times. I miss that intimacy that knows no words but is alive in the shared silence that glues us together. I long for the juicy feeling of being in love, as we were for so long. I feel lonely and empty with one more piece to grieve. How many more pieces will he crumble into? How many more pieces do I have to let go of?

My friends are getting worried about me. I'm losing weight and stress shows clearly on my face. "I don't know how you do it, Susan. I wouldn't be able to," is relayed from friend to friend in one form or another. "You have to take care of yourself. You can't do much for Bob if you become ill, or so stressed you can't function."

When I hear this, it almost feels like they're talking about someone else. Yes, this is intense, but it doesn't often feel intensely awful in the moment. It's only in the light of someone else's perspective that I begin to get the impact of what we're going through. In the day-to-day grappling with caregiving, it feels like I can do this, though I have good days and bad days just like Bob. But there's also a cumulative effect that rears up and whomps me from time to time. It comes from days of repeated irritation over the same issues. It's not being able to deal with someone rationally, not being able to use logic with any meaningful effect. It's having to be manipulative much of the time.

When I reread my journal from the last twelve months all at one go, I see there's a natural numbing process, probably self-preservation, that keeps the intensity sequestered. It's when I read these entries from beginning to end that I feel what others have been seeing for some time.

When we were living with Helen and Lisa, it was the same. In the thick of the pain and challenges of dealing with a teenage drug addict, I knew I was living on the edge, but I was numbed to how torturous it was. It was only when I reread my journals that I saw the gravity of what we were living through. And now here I am again, repeating the pattern.

***

Bob has a perpetual sense that he's going somewhere and is forever packing. The destination varies from America to Bali, to trade shows, to meeting a client, to going home to his parents and his shack in the garden. I find his waist-pack filled with things from the bathroom: his toothbrush, my toothpaste stuffed into a sock, a pair of large scissors, toothpicks, his comb and brush. I silently put them all back. Traveling has been so much a part of our lives that it's no wonder he packs continually. I plunk down on the bed, his belt pack in my hand, and drift off, remembering the year we traveled together early in our marriage.

Chapter Nine
Bali and Beyond

Sweet fragrant
Gardenia blossoms
Spill from garden to house
Overflowing vases
From bush abundant
Candles flicker
In the tendrils
Of a September Bali night

In May 1988 I was back in Ubud designing and producing silver jewelry while Bob tied up loose ends on the second phase of a three-part drapery project he was working on in Sacramento, California. We'd quickly sold most of the inventory we'd bought for Savoir Flair and established wholesale accounts with people who trusted our taste and asked us to ship goods to them as we traveled. Our dream was taking flight.

There were big changes in Bali in the six months we'd been gone, with the building boom leading the way. More shops, cafes, and the occasional spa were replacing the shrinking rice paddies. The traffic was as horrendous as ever, the potholes just as treacherous, and the terrorist monkey continued to break free and have her way with the diners at the Lotus Café. Yet, enchanting Bali still shone through.

Now that I was without wheels and my protective White Knight, I chose to stay in town in the narrow rutted lane directly behind the *pasar,* or fresh market. Sania House was a quiet place with small cottages in a luxuriant garden of red hibiscus and heliconia, run by a welcoming family. Other long-term travelers lived there too and we easily created a sense of community.

***

Agung Rai started selling paintings to tourists on Kuta beach when he was a kid. With his natural business acumen, he'd parlayed his earnings to such an extent that he'd become a major art dealer in the Ubud area. I started painting at his gallery in Peliatan along with a group of foreigners, including two women who introduced me to their Indonesian teacher, Wayan Sidakarya. I began private lessons immediately.

I've always loved languages. With every new phrase my experience deepens as people appreciate that I'm at least making an attempt, no matter how badly I tangle the words. It took a month of guffaws for me to realize I was saying, "I'm a river" when I meant to say, "I'm relaxed." Even I had a good chuckle.

Wayan also initiated me into the world of Balinese Trance Dance when he asked if I wanted to go to Kesiman Temple in Denpasar for a special *Calonarang*, a ceremony that happens every two hundred and ten days, the length of a year in the Balinese calendar.

We arrived to a chaos of color. Throngs of people were entering and leaving the temple, passing stalls set up outside selling food and toys, watches, household items, and opportunities at games of chance. Women dressed in multi-colored batik sarongs and lacy *kebaya*, the traditional Indonesian blouse, walked past with pyramids of food offerings balanced on their heads. Inside the walls, men and women sat on the ground, their hands upraised in prayer as the priest's assistants flung holy water over them in graceful arches and handed out soaked rice grains they applied to their throats, temples, and foreheads, and sprinkled over their heads.

Four *Barong* stood quietly behind those in prayer. The Barong is a mythical, cat-like creature, the guardian spirit of the village and a symbol of goodness. Like the lion who dances at Chinese festivals, his costume and mask require two men inside to animate him. His counterpart in the Calonarang is Rangda, an evil witch with long, scraggly hair and pendulous breasts who needs only one man to dance her to life. Together, they represent the balance between good and evil that lies at the heart of the Balinese world.

As the Barong and Rangda danced their opposition accompanied by a drummer, the energy built to a crescendo until several young men leaped up in trance, their arms rigid and outstretched. Their friends tried to restrain them, but they fought with all their might, screaming and shouting. The Barong and Rangda, too, quickly fell into trance, along with a few children and one desiccated old woman. Our attention snapped left, then right, as we tried to keep track of the enchanted ones so we could stay out of their way. One by one they were led to the outer courtyard as bedlam ensued.

Maintaining the balance between good and evil is essential in Balinese culture. However, those in trance were obsessed with the desire to banish evil by killing Rangda. Each of them was given a *kris*, a sharp long-bladed ceremonial knife, but they were impotent against Rangda's power. In frustration, they turned the kris on themselves, thrusting the sharp points into their naked chests and pushing with all their might until their arm muscles strained and the metal blades bent under the pressure. But although the men's faces twisted in anguish and their arms shook with effort, the knives didn't cut. As long as the trance lasted, they were protected by the magic of the Barong.

All the Balinese, including the entranced, circumambulated the courtyard three times and then poured back into the inner temple. Those in trance were escorted, some struggling to break free, others zombie-like, their heads flopped back, barely able to walk. Some of the children were carried stiff as boards.

I asked Wayan why people did this. "It's a purification ceremony, a form of repentance or gratitude," he told me. "If a person prays and God answers the prayer, that person might come to the temple on this day and be taken by trance." He paused for a moment as we watched the priest and assistants move about, liberally sprinkling those in trance with holy water, returning them to everyday life, but leaving them unaware of what had taken place.

"No one knows who will be chosen," Wayan went on. "It's a combination of belief and surrender. While they're in trance, messages are often relayed by the ancestors. They give instructions for ceremonies and offerings."

The last part of the ceremony featured village elders of both sexes, traditionally dressed, dancing three times around the courtyard. Their withered bodies moved gracefully in perfect unison as though they were still young. Pan-like, they followed a priest wafting burning incense and danced to the clang of the *gamelan*, dancing for the Gods, the ancestors, and tradition.

I thanked Wayan for bringing me. It was the beginning of a long-running passion for trance ceremonies, which I shared with Bob as soon as he arrived. Whenever we experienced these sacred trances, it was as though a portal to the Divine opened and we felt the presence of the sacred. We were deeply grateful for being allowed this peek into another world.

***

Finally Bob arrived and after a week of honeymoon interspersed with introductions to new friends, we spent the next month buying and shipping for Savoir Flair. Excited by newly discovered items like hand painted dreamlike masks, we turned shopping and bargaining into a game. We were tickled when we walked away with a dozen hand-painted sarongs of birds and tropical flowers, trying not to grin too broadly, leaving the shopkeeper briskly tapping the newly-earned bills on items around the store in an Asian gesture of good luck. What could be more perfect than being able to do this for a living?

We finally pried ourselves away to continue our travels, starting with a thrilling forty-five minute flight in a small plane to Waingapu, on the eastern end of the island of Sumba.

***

Sumba was clearly not Bali. Mosques took to the airwaves

at sunrise and sunset, chanting praises to Allah and waking us before we were even remotely ready to face the morning. There wasn't a Hindu temple in sight.

Semi-arid and savannah-like, Sumba had deep, river-cut ravines. The only dense green we saw on that end of the island was along riverbanks where the Sumbanese grew their food and lontar palms for animal food and for making *tuak*, an alcoholic brew. They raised strong, sturdy horses, white hump-backed Brahma bulls with long sweeping horns, and water buffalo for plowing the paddies and vegetable fields.

But what the Sumbanese were most famous for was exquisite *ikat* weavings. No sooner had we checked into our hotel, as far from a mosque as possible, than Kabobo arrived at our door with ikat and old beads. His kind, patient eyes soon had us melting, ready to hand over our wallets in an instant, but in a show of self-control we decided to look around before we bought. We knew what suckers we were for kind eyes that blinded us to good business sense.

The next day we took a bus to Rende, relearning the Southeast Asian bus system of drive-around-for-an-hour-to-find-passengers before departing on a thirty-minute trip. We tried to be patient and appreciate the service this offered the public rather than being annoyed at the inefficiency.

Rende, a traditional village with high-peaked thatch or corrugated-metal roofed houses, is known for some of the best weaving on Sumba. It also has another attraction: huge, ornamental gravestones center stage in the middle of the community. The oldest are massive, dove-gray monoliths supporting enormous rock slabs. Some have three to four foot tall rectangular stone tablets atop the slab, carved with animal, insect, plant, and people motifs. Death on Sumba is the most important event in life. The same motifs are woven into the famous ikat, telling stories of ancestors as well as the daily life of those still earthbound.

Marapu, the much-revered ancestral spirits who inhabit the peaked roofs of houses, watch over the community, protecting and influencing the living. They have to be recognized and venerated through traditional rituals done in prescribed manners or they could raise havoc. Even repairing a house requires the proper ceremony to appease the Marapu. A strong sense of community keeps the whole mechanism functioning.

Ikat weavings play an important role. They are not only worn, but used ceremonially. The best accompany the dead to life in the hereafter. Rende produces some of the most bold and intricate pictorial ikat in Indonesia using time-consuming natural dyes from locally grown and harvested plants. To speed up production, some villages had gone to using chemical dyes, so we knew we had to beware.

Armed with a letter of introduction from Verra at Arts of Asia, we approached Rombu Juliana, the queen of Rende. Bob and I were shy and nervous, but Juliana brightened when she read the letter and invited us for a cup of tea on her veranda once we'd declined her offer to chew betel nut. After tea and a chat, Rombu's wares were brought out. It was then that we realized we were out of our league and the weavings were out of our price range. We were embarrassed that we'd taken up her time. In the end we bought only one small, but delicately woven, scarf.

On our way out of the village a young man accosted us, showing us a beaded lime container like the ones we'd seen for sale at Arts of Asia. Used with betel nut, it still had remnants of lime or calcium hydroxide inside. "It belonged to my mother. She died twenty years ago," he insisted, pulling at our heartstrings. We couldn't resist the story or the container. It joined our collection.

Betel nut chewing has been practiced for thousands of years from Asia to the Pacific. It's offered to guests as a courtesy as a drink would be offered in the West. An areca nut is thinly sliced and folded into a betel leaf with a sprinkling of powdered lime. When chewed, it gives a sensation of heightened awareness and stimulation, but it tastes horribly bitter to the uninitiated, and turns teeth and gums bright red, and the resulting liquid must be spat out, not swallowed. Pavement stains in Sumba were telling signs of its popularity.

***

The next morning we slept in, hoping to sidestep the sellers, but no such luck. Kabobo was back, with six others in tow, and all had patient, kind eyes. There must have been a course there in how to master this look while wresting open a foreigner's pocketbook. We bought a horn and polished wood rice container, sure that it was new in spite of being assured it was old.

Kabobo took us to his home in the small village of Prailiu to see some, 'authentic old pieces'. Grass mats were brought out for us to sit on, betel nut was offered and politely declined, and the whole village gathered, crushing in on us until we felt suffocated. A two-hour bargaining session ensued for rice pots, ikat, beaded lime containers, old beaded necklaces, and a gold-washed silver pendant known as a *mamuli*. We were gambling at this point, buying things that spoke to us, but not really knowing what was authentic and saleable or what prices we should pay.

We stumbled back to the hotel dazed, hot, and tired, only to be greeted by more sellers milling about outside our room. We felt like shark food. The group trailed us to a restaurant where they sat at adjacent tables trying to sell as we ate while we tried to ignore them. Then they followed us back to the hotel. We shut the door for a rest and finally ventured out refreshed, hoping they'd given up and gone home, but no, there they were, all patient and kind-eyed.

An old man charmed me into believing the crocodile-shaped rice pot he was offering was his father's and was very precious to him. One red betel-stained tooth protruded from his mouth as his basset hound eyes implored, "Trust me trust me, this pot is old." I'm that sucker born every minute. Of course the pot wasn't old, but it had charm and we really liked it, and in the end didn't care if it was old or new.

"Maybe later," we'd said earlier to a man who was now waiting for us. We felt we owed it to him to at least have a look, even though we were already out of money and borrowing from the hotel owner until we could get to the bank the next day. We bought his ikat on a promissory note.

***

Buzzing down the road to the western end of Sumba on a

rented motorcycle, we came to a stretch of twists and turns and crossed a line from dry to lush. We were now on the verdant side of the island. After cruising through a mountainous pine forest we started to see clusters of traditional houses with high-peaked roofs that dipped down low, almost obscuring the verandas, giving shade and privacy and the sense that the house was all roof. The houses stood on tall posts, allowing people to walk and work under them or keep livestock out of the sun.

The next day we cruised the countryside with its hills, dales, mountains and stands of trees, very different from dry, eastern Sumba. Herds of water buffalo with white egrets perched on their gunmetal gray hides grazed along the roadside and young boy herders waved when we passed.

We came upon a large group of people, the men in sarongs folded to mid-thigh with the end piece hanging down between their legs almost touching the ground. Stuffed in their belts were long, wooden, sheathed knives with carved horn handles. Bright red scarves wrapped around their heads completed their ensembles. The women, less colorful, were still elegant in hand woven dark blue or black sarongs with aprons around their waists. Almost everyone smiled at us, revealing betel-stained teeth.

Three sacrificed water buffalo lay on the grass in a circle and a framed photo of a young man was on display. We'd come upon the funeral of a university student who'd been killed in a motorbike accident on Bali, where he'd been going to school. After the ceremony, in which he was sent off with the best ikat, betel nut, ornaments, and spirits of water buffalo to make his new life comfortable, he'd take his place with the Marapu. But with his death, the new hope of the family had been extinguished.

***

"Are you perhaps looking for old things?" a shriveled, leather-skinned man wearing the national Muslim cap asked as we made our way back to the hotel. We followed him to his house, and then through a darkened hallway to a storeroom crammed with artifacts. Feeling as if we'd found Sinbad's treasure, we were wide-eyed with delight, but it was twilight and swarms of mosquitoes drove us out with a promise to return in the morning. We went to to sleep that night with sugarplums and rice pots dancing in our heads.

The next day, Mr. Hamil helped us go through his storeroom, extracting items for us to consider in daylight, and we ended up with carved thread winders used in the weaving process, woven rice containers, primitive sculptures in stone and wood, more beaded lime containers, and a drum. We were so pleased with our bounty that we didn't even consider how we'd haul these things back to Waingapu on the motorcycle the next day.

Back on the eastern end of the island we had one more day to explore and make last minute purchases. Kabobo presented us with hand woven scarves, touching us with his generosity.

The S. S. Kelimutu, an inter-island ferry to Kupang on the island of Timor, was taking on passengers when we arrived at the harbor the next morning with our over-stuffed bags. We found a place on deck, sharing a table with Ingrid, a German transplant living in Australia, who was friendly and, while rather opinionated, a wealth of information about Sumba and its culture.

Adjacent to us sat an older woman writing letters, and obviously thoroughly enjoying herself, laughing as she was writing. A good-looking younger man popped in to check on her now and then, his camera ready for action.

For no apparent reason, Ingrid picked up a full ashtray in front of her and plunked it down on the letter writer's table. Then Thud! The letter-writer pointedly re-plunked the ashtray back on our table. Flicking her eyes towards the other table, Ingrid said, "Some people are so self-centered!" eliciting, "How rude!" from the letter writer.

We didn't know it then, but this was our introduction to Gill Marais, who was to become a life-long friend. Perhaps if we hadn't spontaneously jumped ship when it stopped at Ende, on the island of Flores, rather than going on to Kupang, as was our original plan, that friendship wouldn't have been born.

At Ende, a swarm of small boats came out to greet the ship and ferry us to the dock. A rusting hulk just under the surface made it impossible for the larger ship to dock. Bob took most of the bags, leaving me with my backpack. Stepping into a bobbing boat with exposed ribs and a sloping bottom, my fear switched to high alert, especially when there was no room for Bob on my crowded boat. My heart was pounding furiously. Two young Florinese women, university students home on holiday from Jakarta, sandwiched me between them, patting my hand, and telling me it would all be fine.

As our rocking boat made its way towards an empty space,

vying with the other boats for the number one slot to let passengers off, the bow boatman fell into the drink. A suitcase dropped in just after him, and he deftly snagged it with his toes before it could sink, garnering him applause.

As our boat neared the dock, I wanted to be the last to climb the ladder, but unfortunately I was sitting in the number one position. Before I knew what was happening, I was up the ladder with my bag deposited on the dock beside me, trying to catch my breath.

Casual Bob sat out in the passel of boats watching the chaos and waiting his turn. As he emerged laden with his backpack, a tube bag full of our purchases, and the drum slung over his shoulder, the crowd cheered him for his agility in maneuvering over the ribs of the bobbing boat and making it up the ladder.

In those intoxicating days of adventure I had no idea that Bob, my protector, the man who took charge of the practical and physical dimensions of our journey, whose humor and light buoyed me up when I got scared, would reverse roles with me when Alzheimer's entered our world.

***

Sleepy Ende had little appeal for us. After checking out the town, idyllic beach, and a primitive village four kilometers along the coast, we were ready to move on. We noticed dullness in people's eyes that we hadn't seen on Sumba, so we asked a young man who spoke passable English why this might be. "My mother and father are sister and brother," he told us. "When the Christians came to convert us, they tried to discourage this practice, but it's our tradition."

With our bags secured on the roof of a small bus, we were directed to sit in the back next to two betel-chewing ladies. I moved my daypack and feet out of splatter distance. When Bob went out to check on our bags I had to fight off man who wanted his seat, and wished I had better command of the language so I could be more diplomatic.

By the time the bus left it was jammed, but we still cruised around for the customary hour picking up goods and people. I counted twenty seats and forty-five passengers, with six of them riding outside the bus, hanging onto the grab bar at the doorway. Almost every man was smoking.

Three hours and thirty-five miles later along a bumpy road, we pulled into Wolowaru in central Flores. This rambling village is the nearest settlement to the mysterious, three-colored lakes in the crater of the Kelimutu volcano. No one knows why each lake is a different color, or why the colors change from time to time.

From Wolowaru, we joined two Englishwomen for a trek to Nggela, a village perched above the sea twelve kilometers away that was known for its weaving. The hot, dusty walk, steep in places, shaded in others, yielded breathtaking vistas of the undulating landscape and occasional glimpses of the coast below. Around one bend we came upon a towering, many-branched kapok tree in full fluffy splendor. "How many mattresses do you think it'll yield?" wondered Bob. This is what we'd been sleeping on for the last month.

Approaching the village, we were impressed with the tidiness of its fields, fences, and houses. As soon as they spotted us, the citizens literally came running towards us bearing weavings. Their ikat was less dramatic than on Sumba, with darker, more muted colors and smaller designs, more delicate and subtle. We sat in the shade and looked at the wares, but the prices were fixed and there was no room to bargain for these top quality weavings. Again, we only bought one as the gamble seemed too big for our small budget.

Our attention was pulled away by chanting and wailing coming from one of the houses where a funeral for an eight-year-old boy was in progress. This was the third funeral we'd come upon in two weeks and all had been for young people. It left us feeling somber. Life in these islands was hard, medical treatment scarce, working hours long and physically challenging.

Kelimutu, with its magical lakes, apparently wasn't meant for our eyes. The car and driver we'd arranged for the next morning didn't turn up, and we both had such tender blisters that there was no way we could put on sport shoes, let alone trek to the volcano. We packed and took a long, hot bus ride to Maumere on the north coast.

At the bus station on the outskirts of Maumere, a private *bemo* driver tried to charge us ten times the local price. We were hot and tired, and yelled at him, then turned in a huff and walked away, not having a clue how we'd get into town. A group of children took us to the city *bemo* stop just around the corner where we got close to the local price for the ride into town. We checked into the Maiwali Hotel.

A commotion woke us at midnight as luggage was dragged down the hall.

"This room is filthy! I can't stay here!" screamed an angry woman "And you want twice the price you quoted us on the phone?" Bags were dragged back out. The door slammed. We went back to sleep.

The next morning, the staff told us our room cost twice what we'd been quoted. Miffed, we packed and checked out, refusing to pay more than the agreed amount. Nearby, we got a bigger, better room for almost the same price. Maumere was beginning to grate on us.

That evening at the new hotel, familiar faces from the S.S. Kelimutu, emerged from a room. The letter writer, Gill, and her man, Geoffroi, joined us in the lobby where we fell into easy conversation. Photojournalists from Paris with assignments to write articles on Indonesian royalty, they'd been traveling Indonesia for six weeks. He was French, she South African. We learned it was Gill's voice that had woken us at the Maiwali. She was still indignant. During dinner we all expressed the same feeling that there was a spark missing here that was alive and well on Sumba even though both islands shared similar levels of poverty. The empty stares on people's faces disturbed us, making us wonder what had taken away their spirit.

The next morning, after a deliciously intimate time together, Bob and I were ready to 'go home' to Bali. Gill and Geoff had flights to Denpasar the following day and we decided to see if we could change our tickets and leave too.

It was market day, as it is every three days throughout Indonesia. Farmers and suppliers arrived in town loaded with fresh vegetables, chickens, and eggs. The *pasar* was bustling with more energy than we'd seen expended in one spot the whole time we'd been on Flores. We bought papayas and limes for breakfast, and long purple eggplants, greens, bean sprouts, and herbs. We planned to ask hotel staff to cook this bounty for dinner since their veggie repertoire seemed to be limited to carrots and green beans.

Geoff and Gill had also been to the *pasar* and bought tomatoes, celery, and onions. While the kitchen cooked our food, the four of us sat on the veranda making a tomato salad and sharing stories. Locals wandered by, stopping short, not believing their eyes that *bule* actually knew how to make food themselves. Soon we had a crowd four deep pressing in on us, with their hands on the table to steady the crush and their bellies in our faces. We finally asked them to back off, but they were too fascinated to leave. We got a kick out of being the evening's entertainment once again. The kitchen delivered a steaming dish of our eggplant, carrots, tempe, onions, and bean sprouts stir-fried to perfection and slathered with a spicy sauce that I wanted the recipe for.

***

"Is the flight full?" I enquired at the airport. The Merpati agent scrutinized our tickets and added them to a pile on the counter, ignoring my question. It wasn't until we were buckling our seat belts that I felt certain we were leaving. Just after take-off, the pilot announced he was giving us a special treat that day, and circled the three colored lakes set in adjoining deep craters on Kelimutu. That day, one was a deep turquoise, another wine red, and the third black. He circled twice, giving each side of the plane a good look, and we chuckled at the irony of finally seeing the lakes from a bird's eye view.

***

At twilight on my forty-second birthday, the second birthday I'd celebrated on Bali, Bob and I were escorted from our guesthouse bungalow into the garden, where chairs had been set up for a special *Legong* dance to mark the occasion. Geoff and Gill arrived, and with the click of a cassette player, gamelan music filled the evening air. Six little girls, ranging in age from four to ten, entered. They were heavily made up with red cheeks, lipstick, and black curls painted on their foreheads and temples. Their headdresses, adorned with yellow frangipani blossoms and gold-leaf decorations, bobbed in cadence with the choreography as they wiggled their hips to center stage. Barefoot, they were dressed in green sarongs and white chest wraps, both stenciled in gold, leaving their arms and shoulders bare.

By the time they tossed flower petals over the audience, Bob and I were both choked up. I was honored by their performance, and their mother's behind-the-scenes efforts, and tickled at how cute they were. Geoff and Gill had gone through rolls of film.

Many friends came to the party we held later at Café Wayan. Ben, who we'd bought the pelangi jackets from the year before, and who rarely ventured out of his compound, turned up. Our landlords, Sania and Theodora, our painter friend Tom, Agung Rai and his wife, Wayan Sidakarya, plus a few others we'd met along the way came to celebrate too. Geoff and Gill later gave me a photo-reportage of the party and the *Legong* Dance. Bound in a bright yellow, clear plastic cover complete with captions and story line, it was a gift that I've treasured for years.

Geoff and Gill were already sold on the island and vowed to be back, dreaming of building a Bali house. This was also our farewell party. Bob's visa was expiring and we had places to go, people to see, and Savoir Flair to stock.

Chapter Ten
The Subcontinent

There is no goal
On this journey without destination
Only the unraveling of the heart
To reveal the seed of ten thousand sighs
Breathing in beauty and perfection
Breathing out Mystery
Beyond explanation

We arrived late one night, and awoke to a morning that felt like One-Thousand-and-One-Arabian-Nights set in a Lilliputian medieval Europe, all ground up in an Osterizer and poured out at our feet. Kathmandu, Nepal's capital, captivated us instantly. We wandered dung-covered, rocky dirt roads, weaving in and out of dogs, cows, goats and people going about their lives in a warren of ancient buildings on this segment of the old Silk Road. The aroma of Indian spices overlaid a rainbow of other scents from the sublime to the disgusting: sandalwood, carbon monoxide, jasmine, sewage, rose, and rot.

Like enchanted children, we tugged at each other's sleeves to point out miniature three-foot doorways and windows framed by intricately carved wooden trim. "Who lives in these?" we asked each other, "Friends of Gulliver?" Many were shops where almost anything was on offer, including gold and silver, turquoise nuggets, sparkling gemstones, fabrics, marijuana, hashish, or the opportunity to change money on the black market. Our Savoir Flair radar switched on.

In the square by our hotel, an open wall surrounded a stupa with twelve copper prayer wheels on each side. I fell into line with the locals who were spinning them as they whispered the Tibetan prayer *Om Mani Padme Hum*, a mantra with many layers of definition, often translated as "Hail the Jewel in the Lotus". Each turn of a wheel sent this mantra out into the world in benediction. Bob watched for a few minutes, a little self-conscious, then surrendered himself to the turning, and to this adventure that would test our values, broaden our perspectives and smack us in the head a few times.

Learning to be an objective observer seemed to be the theme superimposed over this Asian odyssey. Stepping over blood running from a butcher's stall, filthy, snotty-nosed children, and lepers displaying their rotted stumps, we learned to accept the reality of life lived close to the bone rather than make judgements. These scenes touched a fear cringing in a corner of my mind that I might one day be forced, through some incomprehensible circumstance, to live like this. In Nepal I found myself looking more intently, and with more compassion, at scenes that previously would have repulsed me or had me recoiling in fear.

We found three Thangkas, sacred Buddhist paintings colored with natural stone pigments such as lapis lazuli, jasper, and cinnabar, all ground into fine powders and mixed with a binder. These pigments are applied to stretched cotton canvas in prescribed and detailed designs of sacred geometry that tell stories of the Buddha and his insights. We excitedly added them to our growing inventory.

***

After exploring Kathmandu and its environs for two weeks, we made a shattering, seven-hour bus trip to Pokhara to trek in the Himalaya. Exhausted, we took the first tout's offer of a room and found Annapurna One, Two, Three and Four, and Machapuchare, the fishtail mountain, all at least twenty thousand feet high, smack dab in front of us. When veiled by the saturated, crisp morning air, they looked faint and mirage-like. As the oxygen molecules warmed up, the air brightened, revealing opalescent colors that morphed from cold, whitish gray into soft pinks, peaches, yellows, and blues.

Bob, ever Mr. Practical, went about organizing trekking permits and finding a porter to carry our bags for an eight-day tea-house trek, where we'd sleep in basic rooms with or without doors or glass in the windows and with toilets often a block away.

On the hiking trail, deep-throated clanging would demand our attention. We'd be facing a mule train coming towards us, tinkling their mountain music that warned us to step aside. The animals were bedecked with tall, wool plumes and forehead decorations woven into floral designs using every color the wool company produced. Occasionally, the flash of an intricately woven Tibetan rug flung across a donkey's back startled us. We passed these trains all day long with stout horses, donkeys, and mules carrying everything and the kitchen sink. We also passed many porters on foot with men, women, and children all hefting heavy loads.

After eight days of oohing and ahhing our way through the mountains, we descended again to Pokhara, high on the beauty we'd seen and the accomplishment of doing the trek.

***

"Bye-bye Pokhara! Bye-bye Nepal. Heeello India!" At the Nepali-Indian border town of Sunauli, we boarded a nearly empty Indian bus that stayed that way for the first twenty miles. Then, at stops along the way, people jammed on with sacks of this and boxes of that, which they plunked down in the nearest available space, usually the aisle close by the door. Everyone who followed had to either step on or over the obstacles while the owners looked on disdainfully. It was clear that we were complete novices in India, which felt so different from laid back Nepal.

We hadn't come to India on a spiritual quest. We just wanted to touch its history, meander through its World Heritage sites, meet its people, and eat its food. And we hoped to find crafts to add to Savoir Flair's inventory. But the spiritual quest herded us in her direction.

We'd been mesmerized by the Taj Mahal and camel trekking in Rajasthan. We'd been dumbstruck by motor vehicles sharing four to six lane roads with horse, donkey, camel, and bullock carts, along with free-roaming goats, pigs and piglets, burros, cows, dogs, and the odd water buffalo. Monkeys leaping across rooftops tickled our funny bone while the smell of multi-species dung often hung in the air. This menagerie of animals made us smile. But the spiritual quest wormed its way through all this and caught us off guard in Varanasi.

The great Ganges River was shrouded in mist as the sun cleared the horizon, struggling to penetrate the gloom. We drifted in a small boat parallel to the bathing *ghats* on shore. The measured dip-dip of oars was hypnotic. It was festival day, and the shore-length stairs leading into the water were jammed with pilgrims who'd come for a ritual dip in the sacred waters. The women submerged fully dressed in saris, the fabric fanning out Desdemona style. The men stripped down to shorts or jock straps, held their noses, and hunkered down under the water, blowing bubbles. Everyone seemed oblivious to the cold; joy and ecstasy warmed them from within.

The burning ghats further downriver were quiet. The previous night several death processions had passed by. We'd seen the bodies bathed in the river first, and then put on tall log pyres, the men covered in white cloth, the women in colorful saris. More wood was put over them. We'd watched the eldest son, barefoot and clad in white with his head shaved, circle the pyre five times, once for each of the body's elements - fire, water, ether, air and earth - then set the logs alight and leave the tending to the Doms, the caste responsible for cremations. A local man had told us, "Eighty to ninety bodies are burned here every day. It's an honor to die along the banks of the Ganges. It assures freedom from the wheel of reincarnation."

Death, so obviously a part of life in Asia, seems hidden in the West, as though it's a mistake, and old age is a disease to be cured. Bob had bumped up against death a few times in his life. He was three when his dad climbed with him in his arms up the highest diving tower in Long Beach, California. Somehow, little Bobby got loose and went off the end of the board, plunging ten meters into the pool. Everyone froze as the lifeguard pulled his limp body out. His parents got to him just as he took a breath. But it didn't dissuade him.

He told me as we gazed out at the river, "I loved to dive, whether it was off a high board or free diving in the ocean. I was in my twenties, when an auxiliary air supply was first introduced, before there were formal diving tanks. A buddy and I hooked ourselves up to airplane oxygen tanks. I was down about a hundred and fifty feet when I breathed right through my reserve and couldn't find my friend. I started up towards the light and screamed the last of it so I wouldn't take a breath. I was weak as a kitten when they hauled me back into the boat." He shuddered with the recollection. "It happened again another time, when the first scuba tanks were introduced. I never thought I'd live to be this age."

Bob's recollections silently affected both of us in a way we couldn't voice. We both felt stirred up inside so it felt natural to abandon sightseeing and train to Bodhgaya where the Buddha attained enlightenment twenty-five hundred years ago sitting under the bodhi tree for which the town is named. Most Buddhist countries are represented here with monasteries of their own.

We'd done a weekend meditation retreat in Kathmandu and the teacher there had told us about a ten-day silent vipassana retreat in Bodhgaya. We'd applied, not knowing if room was still available. Since this was a new addition to our travel itinerary, we weren't attached either way. We'd wanted to see Bodhgaya anyway, and found when we arrived that we'd been accepted.

We bought warm blankets from Tibetan sellers and gathered snacks to hide in our rooms, fearing that the traditional two meals a day wouldn't be sufficient. When we stopped for a drink in town, sitting at a communal table, Bob ordered a 'special lassie' and after a few sips said, "This tastes really weird, kind of like new mowed lawn."

"Special means they put marijuana in it," our tablemate informed us. "Perfectly legal here."

"A great way to kick off a retreat!" Bob mused.

As usual, he coasted along happily, giving me plenty of space since we were housed in separate quarters in the Thai monastery. Nothing seemed to faze Bob during the retreat while I went so deeply into pain, sadness, guilt, and anger that I feared for my sanity.

It started on day one during a morning meditation when tears welled up. I tightened against them, trying to stay in control. No specific thoughts caused the tears. They just came on their own and then thoughts formed around them. I felt so separate and alone.

By day two I was crying through most meditations, both walking and sitting. My senses were also becoming hyper-alert. During walking meditations I could feel a 'space' that surrounded me as though I extended about eighteen inches beyond my skin. I also sensed the space of other people, or even the trees that I passed. It was as if their energy field had an elastic quality, as though the fields reached out to each other magnetically, then pulled apart to breaking point like gum on the sole of a shoe. I experienced the sponginess of the earth, even on cement. Nothing seemed solid. This merging of energies continued through most of the retreat. I tried to observe it and not analyze it or make it appear important. I felt I was learning to walk.

A few nights later I couldn't sleep and went for a moonlight stroll. Feeling the energies of the trees, I realized that I had no unique energy field. For forty-two years I had carefully guarded a boundary that didn't exist! It's a shared energy field. Sadness welled up, and suddenly I distrusted the whole process. *Maybe this is all garbage, imaginings, ego, desire for glorification.* I didn't trust myself to let go, just be in the moment, and observe what was going on.

I was living a dream life with my soulmate, deeply in love, and yet I was spending a lot of the retreat crying and I didn't know why. Sometimes I felt I'd burst with this tenderness of spirit. I wanted to walk gently on the earth. Where did this sensitivity come from? Then the flipside would erupt and I'd explore anger. Pain, sadness, and anger slid one into the other.

Fortunately, there were experienced teachers to talk with to keep those of us in need on the right footing. The retreat leader told me, "In light of the anger, I'd say you were probably held in check pretty tightly as a kid. What you're experiencing is old wounds healing in a natural way." He told me it wasn't necessary to know the specifics about the wounding, only to let it out and feel what the tears brought.

The insights those painful days uncovered were an annuity that came due when Alzheimer's entered our world. I was seeing what a great healer awareness is. I was learning not to fear anger and the underlying pain but to just observe, and in that watching, change would happen on it's own. Just observing would allow me to consciously right myself more quickly and to understand my feelings. The lessons learned at Bodhgaya sustained me when life became close to unbearable. The idea of staying with pain and sadness, not analyzing it, not avoiding it, but simply experiencing it, would help me endure the pain of losing my soulmate to this disease.

***

For a while, the spiritual journey trumped buying for Savoir Flair. After the retreat we went to Puri for a month of yoga. Then, between visits to historical sites in the sweltering pre-monsoon heat, we were guided to two spiritual teachers in the South. While these were interesting experiences and we sensed both were authentic sages, we didn't feel drawn to either of them as personal teachers. Meanwhile, gemstones were quietly calling our names.

With only a week left on the subcontinent, we trained to Jaipur, famous for gems, where our Italian friend Mauro had recommended a dealer he used. We sipped sweet, hot, milky tea with Zahire, discussing what we'd learned browsing in shops in Nepal and India, and what stones we thought we'd like to buy. He offered sound advice, steering us towards stones most easily sold. We soaked up his knowledge and left Jaipur with packets of amethyst, garnet, black sapphire, lapis, onyx, moonstone and other semi-precious stones.

Back in Kathmandu it was pelting rain as we made our way to the jeweler's shop where we'd left our purchases for safekeeping five months earlier. Down to our last sixty dollars in cash, we were both jittery when our last traveler's check proved un-cashable. But this time the anxiety and fear that had dogged me for years became a point for meditation. I watched it arise and saw where it settled in my body. This helped me feel a modicum of control. In a moment of clarity, I saw this whole journey with fear as an exciting challenge. I discovered that underneath it lay excitement.

American Express in Bangkok came to our rescue and allowed us to buy more traveler's checks, giving us the means to top up stock for Savoir Flair. We also spent two weeks learning more about gemstones from Mauro, who'd advised us where to buy in Jaipur. He'd been living in Thailand for a few years and invited us to stay with him in a house that seemed luxurious after the places we'd been staying in the previous months. Completely focused on gemstones, he expounded for hours while we became his apprentices, listening to more information than our brains could assimilate.

Our plan was for Bob to return to California to take care of loose ends, prepare for the last of a three part drapery installation and sell some of our inventory while I went back to Bali to produce silver earrings for Savoir Flair. We'd grown so close during the ten-month journey that, knowing we'd be separated for the next seven weeks, I could barely choke out "I love you!" through my good-bye-tears. All those months together should have had me running for alone time, but instead I'd become even more attached to this handsome, generous, caring man.

***

Before moving up to Ubud, I stayed in Kuta for several days to design earrings with some of our Jaipur stones and to be close to the silver factory. I was less confident without Bob and found eating on my own rather lonely.

But back in Ubud, Theodora at Sania House embraced me wildly, an unusual action for a Balinese woman. Grandma was all smiles. The little dancer, Juni, and her friend came and sat on the veranda for a chat. It was like coming home. Everyone, of course, asked about Bob.

"Tom and his daughter are here," Theodora informed me. I left a note for them at their homestay. The same warm welcome awaited me at Kokokan along with an avocado smoothie. "I have a surprise for you," said Ben. "Geoff and Gill are here and they're building a house!"

Geoff was reading on their bungalow's veranda when I tiptoed up and stood in front of him. When he looked up, shock melted into, "Wow! How great to see you!" We caught up quietly, not wanting to disturb Gill, who was napping upstairs.

"I heard someone talking and I thought, There's a nice person downstairs, a very nice person, a very, very nice person." Down she came, engulfing me in yet another embrace. I felt like a love surfer.

Back at Sania's, Tom had left me an invitation for cocktails. He greeted me with a hug, a kiss, and an introduction to Linda, his daughter. It was as though Tom and I hadn't been apart. We yakked for hours until we gave up and went to our rooms for much needed sleep.

A few days later I took the bus south to check on my samples at the silver factory in Kuta. I was disappointed by how little progress had been made.

"Don't worry, Susan, everything will be ready in three days," Talip, one of the brother-owners, assured me.

I was doubtful. I obviously had a lot to learn if I wanted to produce jewelry in Bali. Disheartened, I boarded the bus back to Ubud. A wide-girthed American with a ponytail sat down beside me, his bulk spilling over onto my seat. He was smoking. With a deep sigh I folded my arms across my chest and stared hard out the window. Little did I know that synchronicity was at work, disguised as Trader Rick from Arizona.

Rick, a larger than life character, was full of mesmerizing stories about his travels, reading palms and tarot cards, and dealing in gemstones. In Bali he made carvings of little wizards crafted from fossilized walrus teeth and set with semi-precious stones and crystals. His interest was piqued when I told him about the Jaipur gems.

The next day we met at Lotus Café for the first round of stone viewing. Rick liked what I had so we went back to his place to weigh them on his karat scale. He bought all my remaining moonstones, black stars, most of the lapis, and some of the amethyst. I was wishing we'd bought more stones, but relieved to have made my first sale after an otherwise disappointing day.

I wouldn't realize for several years that this was a life-changing meeting, the seed that sprouted into "World on a

String", the business that would allow us to live our dream for the next twenty plus years.

Three days later, back in Kuta I faced more disillusionment. No work had been done on the samples and the price had increased again for inexplicable reasons. "Before I can place the order, I have to approve the samples," I told Talip.

'Saving face' is an important concept in most of Asia, and when Indonesians 'lose face' they often become passive aggressive or space out as though no one's at home. So when I showed my frustration at the lack of enthusiasm and slow results, instead of my silver order speeding up, it nearly ground to a halt.

It's a difficult lesson for Westerners to learn, but learn it we had to if we were going to be at peace on this island. On my next visit I tried very hard not to show my feelings and Talip's reaction was completely different. "It would be better if the silver curved this way," I said neutrally, pointing to the drawing, rather than saying, "You idiot! Can't you see this is completely different from the design I gave you!" That would have got me nowhere because he'd have been embarrassed about not understanding what I wanted in the first place.

With the production finished only two days before I left Bali, I spent a day at the factory going over the order and rejecting thirty percent because of damaged stones or repairs. Instead of reacting angrily, I simply presented Talip with a bill and deducted the damage from my balance owed. He wasn't happy, but he accepted it.

Some of the workers invited me to eat with them and Talip

joined in, more friendly than before. After changing my attitude, I was treated differently. And I felt better about myself. I was learning the value of silence, observation and opening my heart instead of instantly reacting. I'd get a lot of practice in the years to come.

***

Back in the USA, wrapped in the warmth of my soulmate's love, I got the distressing news that I had several fibroid tumors and they needed to come out. I shouldn't have been surprised since both my mother and sister had hysterectomies for the same reason. Somehow, I'd thought with all my meditation and healthy eating, I wouldn't repeat their fate. I vowed to clean up my act and do everything I could to avoid the knife.

Bob suggested a movie Helen had recommended to take my mind off the nagging news. With its theme of, "Follow your dreams no matter where they take you", we felt "Field of Dreams" was speaking directly to us. Luckily, the third phase of Bob's hotel project was ready to install, and he had other installations after that. I became his assistant to help defray costs. We had a dream to live in Bali with the goal to get back there within six months. We could do this.

Chapter Eleven
Home Again Home Again Jiggity Jig Jig

It's a strange time
Of limbo colored scenes
Of floating end over end
Empty handed and naked
Having impulsively stepped off the cliff
Into the cool clear void
Familiar labels wash away
Growing fainter with each surge of time
Leaving me in momentary terror
Nothing to grasp
No chance to go back
Seeded in this flower of fear
Lies a sense of security
A knowing
That calms me
I have no clue how I will land
When the void drains away
Upright or downtrodden
Shattered or whole
The mystery keeps my fire crackling
The unknown fuels my spirit

A fter eight months in the States, Bob and I were back in our Ubud bungalow at Sania House. Tom had also returned, in spite of his dislike of the building boom that had mutated into a blast. Still enamored with Bali's unique culture, its rice paddy beauty and smiling people, he couldn't seem to let the island go.

While we were gone, Ben had revamped his boutique and transformed the adjacent building into a dazzling gallery of contemporary art. Wiranta, a Javanese pallet knife artist, was painting on site; his paintings were a tumult of color bursting with energy and emotion in layer after layer of rainbow strokes.

I visited one day as he was finishing a large canvas of a man and a boy. The boy's extended hand had a bird of peace hovering over it. When Ben said, "Give the boy the hand of Buddha," something inside of me cringed. My free spirit railed against the idea that someone would want to orchestrate an accomplished artist, and worse, possibly orchestrate me. Now, I can see that Ben was mentoring, but at the time I couldn't see beyond my triggered reaction.

I returned nervously that afternoon with watercolor paintings I'd brought from the States. I was reluctant to show them to Ben because I knew what a stickler he was for quality. But relief washed over me when he not only approved, but by that evening had sold the largest one to Agung Rai, the art dealer whose gallery I'd spent months painting in two years earlier.

Tom popped in and we spent hours with Ben talking art while Wiranta put finishing touches to his piece. Ben stood back, one arm across his chest, the other holding his chin in contemplation. Gently, he approached the artist and whispered his critique.

Wiranta pondered for a few minutes, expressionless, while Tom and I watched, hardly daring to breathe. Then Wiranta decisively put palette knife to canvas and stroked the work to completion.

***

When I brought Geoff and Gill to see my paintings a few days later, Ben told us two other important gallery owners had seen the piece Agung Rai had bought and each wanted to commission me to do one for them. I was getting the attention I'd always dreamed of, but it seemed too good to be true. I feared I'd ruin this opportunity.

I started the first commission the next day. A vision came quickly of a pair of cheetahs running through red and yellow heliconia flowers with a pond of white lotuses in the foreground. I was uniting a common element in my paintings (the cheetahs) with my new life in Bali (the tropical flowers). The preliminary drawing moved along quickly and I transferred it to watercolor paper.

It had been months since I'd held the wooden handle of a fine sable hair brush. I dipped its perfect point into sage green and put color to paper. My body hummed with excitement.

The hours at the gallery were interspersed with continuing Indonesian lessons with Wayan Sidakarya. Bob, a beginner, was studying with Wayan on his own. But while my life was full of art and learning, Bob was going through an identity crisis. He was torn between his love of our life in Bali and feeling guilty that he wasn't being productive. He was clear that he didn't want to hang draperies for the rest of his life, but he didn't have any ideas except Savoir Flair for earning a living, and Savoir Flair, still in its infancy, was an unknown. Low self-esteem gnawed at him, filling his night dreams with anxiety and frustration. Yet he still supported my work even as he struggled to right himself in our new circumstances.

***

While grappling with earning a living in those early Bali days, we still found time to gain a deeper understanding of the culture that surrounded and intrigued us, especially the ceremonies and rituals necessary for Balinese life to function. One afternoon we watched four young Balinese men converge at the side of the road bordering a steep embankment. Dressed in traditional sarongs and sashes, they set out small offering baskets with incense, sprinkled them with holy water, and offered a prayer to the Gods. The night before, a bicycle and a motorbike had collided there. While no one was seriously hurt, the bicycle had ended up at the bottom of the ravine. This small ceremony was mandatory to appease any troublesome spirits that might be lurking along the roadway, and to ease the minds of the people involved in the incident. Without it, bad luck might befall the drivers or their families, or worse, their communities.

As we peeled back her layers, Bali was showing us more of her unseen side. This was 180 degrees different from the life we'd been born into. Geoff and Gill whisked us off to sacred springs where cool holy water cascaded over our skin, blessing us, and hopefully washing away any hidden resistance to our new life. Tom took us on walks through the rice paddies to temples in small villages.

At one of our favorites, the Temple of the Navel of the World, just northeast of Ubud, Dewa Ketut Arta, the resident *mangku*, or temple priest, proudly showed us fourteenth century artifacts: a lingam and yoni, a holy water vessel and various sculptures. Dewa came from a long line of temple priests, and giggled like a boy while he was giving us a tour of the grounds and telling us about his three wives and six children. "Each wife has her own room, but they all eat together," he told us proudly. "I sleep with each for a week and they all get equal money." He made it sound like one big happy family. Polygamy had been a tradition in Bali for centuries, but was slowly fading out as modernization took hold and women gained more independence.

The Temple of the Navel of the World was no ordinary temple. Dewa lowered his voice to tell us, "Two mysteries happen here." We leaned in, listening intently. "Sometimes, during a ceremony, a sacred silver cup fills with red, yellow, or clear water. The red portends evil. The other two are benign."

Then there was the seven-hundred-year-old spring, now just a dry depression in the tawny-colored earth. Dewa told us that from time to time he put an offering in the bottom, and after about an hour it disappeared, then reappeared on a beach on Nusa Penida, a small island just off the east coast of Bali. This link brought pilgrims from Nusa Penida to Dewa's temple.

Bob and I found these stories, trance, and the other magical facets of Bali fascinating. We took Dewa's stories in, accepting that if he and the temple congregation believed them, then they were true for them. These views into a different way of living opened us to a world of possibilities much broader than we'd imagined. Bob wasn't able to verbalize how this was changing him, but I could see him relaxing into concepts he would have tossed off as impossible in the West.

***

I started work on the second commission. My pieces took weeks to execute, with layer over transparent layer of color building up to a final depth of hue that isn't possible with one layer of watercolor. In the course of creating a painting, I often tossed and turned in the night in a whirlpool of ideas, colors, and emotions. My mind couldn't find the off switch and I'd lie awake for hours, but somehow I'd wake in the morning with renewed energy. Then, as the painting neared completion, I'd get the jitters that I'd ruin it and all that time would be lost.

Working on that second commission, images came to me in visions, dreams and words. These images seemed to come through me rather than from me and I tried not to question them, but simply to organize them into harmonious composition and color. Gradually, the painting became a powerful image of a cheetah woman with a shield and amulets looking into a mirror so you saw her back as well as her frontal reflection. She was a warrior.

The day of reckoning came. My stomach fluttered and my hands incessantly rubbed the fabric of my skirt as Ben stood back and took in the two new pieces. He liked the first one, with the cheetah running through tropical flowers, which I thought was fine, but safe because the elements in the painting were real, just juxtaposed into a dreamlike scene. But I'd taken a chance on the second piece in merging the woman with the cheetah.

Ben studied it. "It doesn't flow. It's too tight." He turned away, dismissing the painting.

Crushed, I couldn't hear his compliments on the first painting; I could only hear his rejection of the second. I tried to appear unfazed, but inside I despaired. I felt an old, familiar pattern repeating itself: I'd get a great opportunity but couldn't quite grab hold of it and it would fall through my fingers. Something inside clicked as I remembered a pattern of dreams in which I'd win a jackpot or find a treasure, be excited by the prospect and the possibilities and get all revved up, but then it would turn rancid or I'd never get to keep it. I left the gallery asking myself how I could change this pattern.

When I came home, I took one look at Bob and knew something was wrong. He was sitting very still in a bamboo chair on the veranda, holding his side.

"David and I were buying wood carvings in a village up north," he said haltingly. "We filled a duffle bag and David slung it over his shoulder. We tried to take a shortcut back to town. But it turned into a dirt track and then narrowed to mud." Bob winced. "We weren't going very fast, maybe just five miles an hour, inching our way down, when I lost control of the bike in a slurry of slop. David landed on me full force with the carvings. I heard a snap." He sucked in a painful breath. "I have one or two broken ribs."

I wanted Bob to go to a doctor, but he didn't trust Bali's unsophisticated medical establishment. It was common expat knowledge that it was best to leave Bali if you had anything serious. Anyway, he'd had broken ribs before and knew there was nothing to do but let them heal. He was a grin-and-bear-it sort of man, a true Taurus. "It only hurts when I laugh. Or lay down. Or lose my footing," he said. Only.

In spite of Ben's rejection I returned, although now less confident, to the gallery at Kokokan to work on another painting. I had all my materials there, and leaving felt cowardly.

A new painter, Pravit, was in residence, a young watercolorist whose work reminded me of Andrew Wyeth doing Thai village scenes. He was Ben's newest acolyte.

I listened to Ben's suggestions on the direction he'd like to see me take and spent the next four days doing a preliminary drawing. I knew Ben had my best interests at heart. He wanted me to succeed in the Southeast Asian art world. But I also knew I had to trust my intuition. On the one hand, Ben was taking me under his wing, mentoring and guiding me, and I so wanted to listen to him and to please him. But old triggers kept getting pulled.

In the past I'd let myself get emotionally seduced by men who appeared to me as authority figures. I respected them and their knowledge. In those relationships I'd kowtowed, walking self consciously around them, trying to please them, and ended up losing the sense of who I was. I didn't want this to happen again.

My paintings were an expression of my inner vision. When Ben suggested changes, I felt as though he was stabbing me. He was pushing me to paint men, but I didn't have a feeling for the male figure. I tried to conform and drew a man swimming underwater, tattooed with ikat designs and playing with a dolphin. I tried to talk myself into believing this was the right path, but a creeping emptiness spread inside my chest. Ideas stopped coming and I froze, unable to draw for days.

***

Helen came to Ubud on tour with a well-known spiritual teacher and we were invited to some of the events. Her life had settled down in the last year, with Lisa continuing her education at university. Lisa had also joined Santo Daime, a Brazilian religion, and had traveled to Brazil, learning Portugese and immersing herself in the religious practices. In some ways it seemed she'd traded her drug addiction for a religious one, but at least she seemed stable and happy.

Most of Helen's group were interested to know how we came to live in Bali and found it fascinating that we'd give up the familiarity and security of American life. They saw us as courageous, but to us it just felt natural.

Bob hit it off with a couple in the group who owned a store in Massachusetts called 'Heaven and Earth'. They were taken with Balinese handicrafts, but needed an agent to buy and ship during the year. Bob volunteered, and soon had a new lilt to his step in spite of his still-painful ribs.

Helen's roommate fell in love with *Cheetah Woman*, the painting Ben had rejected, and bought it without reservation and without quibbling over the price. My creativity revived and I started drawing again. After much soul-searching I concluded that, though I could learn from Ben, I also had to maintain my integrity and my sense of self. I knew Ben had a lot to teach, but my real job was to develop the self-confidence to know what was right for me, and to be able to distinguish what nurtured my work and what didn't.

***

One day while I was painting at Kokokan, our friend Penny walked in. We'd met a couple of months earlier and she occasionally treated us to ice cream, telling us, "No worries, I'm fabulously wealthy. I have a job!" Penny worked as production manager for a handicraft import business, and she had a wicked sense of humor. She told animated stories of Caribbean living, travels on the hippy trail, and life as a free spirit while we sat on steps in the center of town licking and crunching chocolate-dipped ice cream bars, catching up on news, and watching Ubud go by. On our visa runs to Singapore, Penny sent us with a small icebox and forty dollars to buy cheese at Cold Storage Supermarket since the only cheese available on Bali was processed. She always compensated us with some of the booty. Now she needed a different kind of help.

"My friend Wendyl has just put her back out. She's desperate for a masseuse." Penny looked at me expectantly.

"Penny, I don't feel I'm experienced enough to work on someone who's hurting. I'm afraid I'll make her worse."

Bob walked in as we were talking. "I'll go," he volunteered. We'd taken the same massage course in California two years earlier.

As Bob approached Wendyl's bungalow, a man on a neighboring veranda called out, "Hi! I'm Danny. I do fossil ivory carvings."

Bob said, "I've been looking for you! I'll be back," and

headed up the path to Wendyl's house. He worked with her until she felt relief and then went back to Danny's.

Bob had seen fossil tusk carvings that were very different from those Trader Rick was doing and had been wanting to find the source for Heaven and Earth. Danny had a workshop with a team of expert Balinese carvers. He invited Bob up to the nearby town of Tampaksiring to see the operation. Bob wanted my artist's eye along to help him pick the pieces.

I was immediately drawn to the carvings and the themes. Some of the designs were inspired by the paintings of Susan Boulet, an artist I knew in California. The carvings were archetypal: powerful images of women with owls, eagles, and wolves, and goddesses from ancient cultures. Like my paintings, they told stories. We bought a half dozen to send to Massachusetts and a few for Savoir Flair, but I had ideas for other images I wanted to see carved. I envisioned them beaded into necklaces using the collection of beads we'd bought on our travels.

Bob and Kathy were not as enthusiastic about the carvings as we were. They ordered a few, but not the quantity I'd been sure they would want, so we went to Danny with my ideas and commissioned him to carve designs for us. I couldn't wait to get started beading.

***

Following Ben's suggestion that I work with male figures, I finished a painting with a blue man seated on a Persian rug, his back three-quarters to the viewer, and a pool in front of him with a watery image of a female face. Lying at his side was a Javanese shadow puppet: Arjuna, the Hindu warrior in the epic Bhagavad-Gita. The colors were rich and the composition simpler than my previous work, which tended to leave no empty spaces. Everything was usually filled with design and pattern. I tried to convince myself that I liked this painting, and there were parts of it I did like, but it really wasn't me.

With the completion of this piece, I moved my painting materials home. I was working on another composition Ben was suspect of. It had a woman lying down with her arm stretched over her head. She was dressed in a mauve silk blouse, the sensuous, soft folds almost alive. This is what I liked to paint. I was torn between guilt over leaving Kokokan and a sense of relief that I was painting at home.

I continued to visit the gallery and have long talks with Pravit, who was using Ben's direction to the fullest. His painting career blossomed. I started to feel I'd missed a rare opportunity. The previous months had been a dark tunnel of soul-searching without a torch. I vacillated between feeling that I'd overcome my demons and feeling they'd overcome me.

Bob was happily buying stock for Heaven and Earth and Savoir Flair, always on the lookout for new and interesting pieces, always regaling me with stories of people he'd met along the way. His trips to Tampaksiring to check on our orders with Danny were amusing, as each time Danny spoke at great length about how he had the best carvers on the island and the most creative designs. He exaggerated almost everything, but Bob stayed quiet and observed.

***

To celebrate my forty-fourth birthday we took a ferry

to Lombok, an island to the east of Bali, with three young, vivacious and creative women friends. "It's jammed up jelly tight," Bob groused as we squeezed between the trucks and cars on the parking deck, getting our backpacks caught on mirrors and door handles. The final stretch to the stairs leading to the passenger area required a duck walk under a truck.

The boat was overloaded but there was floor space next to a Lombok policeman, a Javanese truck driver, and a Saudi Arabian taxi driver who'd come to get married. We were getting to know each other when someone shouted, "*Lumba lumba!*" and most of the passengers scurried to the railing.

Out in the rolling swells a few dolphins appeared. Then more arched through the water, circus style, and still more glided in. Soon, thirty gray acrobats were leaping, racing and pirouetting alongside the boat. Dolphins symbolize free spirits to me, and after a recent dream of them circling me in the water, this experience felt electric and synchronistic. There was so much joy in them, in us, and in the air, that tears streamed down my face.

That elation didn't last long, though. A day or two later we were on the tiny island of Gili Air, off the west coast of Lombok, where the well water was briny, and the coffee and tea and showers always salty. I dreamed I was asleep in our hut and something dark and mysterious pulled me down into an abyss. When I awoke, terrified, angst had reappeared. I kept comparing myself to the three young women we were traveling with and seeing them as more confident than I was. A cloud of depression veiled my perception. I wanted to fight against it, but it felt so dense.

Our time together was intense. Our friends told me I was a complainer and a worrier, and one snipped at me in impatience. It was more fodder for 'the peanut gallery', as I'd taken to calling my inner critic.

"Ignore them," Bob told me. "I love you the way you are".

"I love myself. I accept myself unconditionally," I repeated over and over, trying to override the critic and chip away at the boulder in my throat. Our friends' reactions to me were mirroring my fear that I was becoming the person I so desperately didn't want to be. I realized how vulnerable and transparent I was. I wanted to kick sand over these feelings and bury them with acts of courage, courage I didn't think I possessed.

For many years I'd worn the mask of a creative, free spirit, positive and joyous. On Gili Air the mask cracked and splintered off. The mask was who I hoped I was, but with its dissolution I saw my injured parts. This was difficult to accept. *Have I really devolved into a whinger, a nervous Nelly?* I cringed. But something inside counseled: *The only way you can find the real Susan is to stop seeing her through other people's eyes.*

Once back in Ubud, I was grumpy. Everything seemed to irritate me, and poor Bob was getting the brunt of it. I went to the sanctuary of the Lotus Pond when I needed to be alone. I didn't want to inflict myself on anyone, let alone my husband.

But in the dark silence, ideas sprouted. I started painting again. Two Balinese masks came alive on my paper, with a gemstone tear dripping from the female mask's eye onto the male mask below. Large, pink, fully opened lotus flowers framed the masks while a frog dived into a muddy pond below. When I finished *Diving Into Dreamtime*, I took it to Ben.

"Why do I keep torturing myself this way?" I asked Bob on the way to the gallery.

"Because you're still trying to get your father's approval," he answered gently.

Ben stepped back and contemplated the painting for an agonizing couple of minutes. "Surrealism!" he said, as though he didn't know that's what I painted. "I've seen it before." And then he added "Oh, I don't like the subject matter."

Once again I was crushed. But I knew this piece was authentic.

"I can't be one of Ben's craftsmen painting his images. My art is me!" I said fiercely as I collapsed into Bob's arms once we were home.

He held me and let me cry. "All I want is for you to paint what you want. I want to see you blossom, Suz." He looked directly into my eyes, "Making money from your pieces isn't important. We'll make it other ways."

With Bob's support, I kept painting. I was also creating new designs for Danny's carving workshop and beading them into necklaces. They drew such positive comments that I was inspired to continue. When we were out on buying trips for Heaven and Earth or Savoir Flair, we'd easily find semi-precious stone beads in many shapes and colors along with ancient glass beads dug up on Java. We seemed to have natural bead radar that led us to them. That radar stayed with us for years.

Combining beads with the fossil ivory carvings helped satisfy my creative urge. I felt I was painting with these materials, creating textures and harmonies using the same color and composition sense I used in my paintings. The fossil ivory was rich and earthy, varying from white to cream to chocolate to caramel to a rare blue, and finally black. Minerals in the permafrost had created these hues, leaching into the buried tusk over eons on the islands of the Bering Sea.

The Inuit on Saint Lawrence Island are the only people who can legally excavate this fossil material. They also dig through their garbage dumps looking for broken fishhooks, net needles, harpoon heads, and other damaged tools they'd long ago fashioned from it. It tickled me that we were beautifying people's lives with garbage.

Every time we saw the pieces transformed from my two dimensional drawings into bas-relief carvings it felt like Christmas. But although the quality was reasonable, it annoyed me that Danny insisted any design I brought him was his to carve as well. That meant his prices on my images would be cheaper than ours since we paid him a premium to carve at his workshop.

***

Before we knew it, our two-month visa was up and it was time to leave Bali again. We took some of our carvings and necklaces to Bangkok 'just in case'.

In search of a cold drink one afternoon, we happened upon

Harmonique, a quaint, artsy coffee shop in a restored shop-house just around the corner from the General Post Office. After the polluted cacophony of New Road, it was an oasis. The owners, a Dutchman, Jacques, and his Thai partner, Boonma, sat down to chat while we indulged in Boonma's thirst-quenching iced chocolate. They immediately asked about our neckpieces. Bob was wearing one of Trader Rick's wizards on a leather cord with a few antique beads; I was wearing a piece with a woman's face surrounded by an eagle, set with lapis on a string of lapis, amethyst and malachite beads mixed with Balinese sterling silver. Jacques and Boonma couldn't keep their eyes off them.

These two lively, elegant men sold a small amount of selected South East Asian antiques and art pieces in their café. Jacques was the salesman and Boonma the artist, and together they'd created an East-West atmosphere we'd rarely seen in our travels. We spent hours with them over the following week, and before the end of our stay they'd ordered a dozen pieces.

Chapter Twelve
Life's Little Ambushes

Every moment of light and dark
Is a miracle

-Walt Whitman

In the fall of 1991, Bob flew back to America to sell Savoir Flair's inventory while I stayed on Bali producing inventory. I was beading like a madwoman. My third grade report card had come with a teacher's remark: 'Does not use time wisely'. I've been using my time wisely ever since.

The novelty of being on my own soon wore off. It hit me while sketching a new design concept on a coffee-stained napkin in Made's Warung in Kuta. Leo Sayer came on the music system.

'When I need love, I hold out my hands and I touch love...' A lump formed in my throat, obliterating the design idea. 'I never knew there was so much love keeping me warm night and day.' Tears streaked down my face. I'd recorded this song for Bob during our first year together just before I drove alone cross-country selling my paintings at art festivals. 'Miles and miles of empty space in between us...' I felt like an amputee.

It didn't help that Bob's daughter, Michele, was in Bali with her boyfriend, John. They were all over each other, madly in love. I ached to sleep with my soulmate, holding hands throughout the night. I longed for our easy conversation, our silences, and our 'old jeans' comfort.

Back in the States, Bob was losing heart and beginning to doubt we could manifest our dream. I wrote, "I know it's hard for you to keep our vision of making a living with our creations – so don't worry about it. I'll put more energy into creating it and making it work. I know we're meant to live outside the rat race and be who we truly are. Go to comedies, Bob, read funny books and keep laughing so you don't lose the light of our dreams." I listened to a success tape in the evenings, determined to let go of old beliefs and live the life we wanted, but sometimes it felt like two steps forward and one step back.

When I went up to Tampaksiring to check on an order at Danny's, I was disappointed, especially for the price he was asking. Tact, not one of my strong points, flew out the window. "These aren't anywhere near the quality of the first pieces," I moaned. "I'd be embarrassed to show these!"

"Go find your own carvers then!" he growled, and abruptly turned away. I refused to let him see me cry. It wasn't until I was well away from the workshop that I finally broke down.

I sought out Trader Rick. "You don't need Danny! Go see Putu at Goddess. He'll carve for you. Danny doesn't have a corner on the carver market. The Balinese up here have been carving for centuries. They have it in their genes. "

Getting fired by Danny turned out to be a stroke of luck.

Putu was happy to have a new customer, and while working together was challenging at times, we worked through it as my Indonesian improved. I was happy with the results and focussed on designing and beading the finished pieces.

A friend sent me a young Balinese woman, Suarni, to clean house and learn to make necklaces. I only needed her a few days a week, but it was the start of a long relationship. She still works for me today, more than twenty years later. We've seen each other's vulnerable parts, bolstered each other through hardship, and built a deep trust. Like my other long-term employees, Suarni is family.

***

My landlord installed a phone on which I could receive calls but couldn't call out, and the first fax office in Ubud opened. I wrote long letters to Bob, telling him all my news: "The ducks are in the newly shorn paddies quacking and paddling and zipping along the raised paths. They love this rain. The flooded paddies reflect the mood of the sky, grey today, blue yesterday. And Kucing the cat has moved in. I seduced him with cat crunch and now he sleeps on the chair on the upper veranda. He's a poor substitute for you, Bob, but something warm and fuzzy to pet."

Besides producing for Savoir Flair, I'd taken over Bob's job of shipping goods to Heaven and Earth. I pushed myself mercilessly.

***

The Bali monsoon was full on, cloaking the house in dusk all day, making beading difficult. Suarni's young eyes had an easier time of it, but even with stronger light bulbs it was slow going for both of us. Eventually, we had eight pieces finished for Harmonique, Jacques and Boonma's shop in Bangkok. I had such a rush of satisfaction and awe looking at these pieces with their carvings that told stories and beading that led the eye up and down strands of semi-precious and ancient glass beads that I wondered who'd created them. These weren't necklaces for the timid. They were sculptures to wear and be noticed.

I contemplated how my artistic life had changed. Unlike painting, I felt secure in creating jewelry, perhaps because it wasn't all me. I was the conductor and my musicians were the carvers and Suarni. And instead of all the paraphernalia I needed for my style of painting, I could pack my stock and beads, stringing tools and threads, and my twelve ice cube trays into one suitcase.

I used the trays to separate my beads so each indentation held a different size and type of bead. At the supermarket in Denpasar I bought all six on the shelf. Returning two weeks later, I again bought all in stock. But on the next trip there were none. I waited a week and tried again, but left empty-handed. Finally, curiosity and need got the better of me. "When will you have more ice cube trays?" I asked the clerk.

"Oh, finished," she said, looking indifferently past my shoulder at a spot in the distance.

"Yes, I see that, but when will more arrive? Have they been ordered?"

"Oh no, no, not ordered. Someone keeps buying them all."

There had to be some logic there. Perhaps it was too much

bother to order them if they kept selling out. I expanded my hunt to other stores until I had twelve, which seemed almost excessive. Twenty years later I have more than ten times that, all filled with beads in different sizes, shapes, and materials.

My time in Bali was coming to an end. Doing this all on my own had been an initiation, and I realized I could run Savoir Flair by myself if necessary. Feeling empowered, my new motto (borrowed from a book title) was 'Feel the fear and do it anyway.'

***

Back in the States, Bob and I focused on selling our work. The desire to return to Bali propeled us on a road trip in search of new customers and materials. The journey led us to Quartzsite, Arizona where Trader Rick had told us there was a show he did each January. There was also a bigger, more professional one in Tucson every February.

Only two thousand people officially lived in the dusty, desert backwater of Quartzsite with its truck stops and fast food outlets, but the population swelled to hundreds of thousands in the winter when the 'snow birds' migrated in their campers and RVs from colder climes. The desert was dotted with makeshift campsites nudged between the saguaro cactus and scrub.

Bob and I pulled into the burgeoning town, excited by the prospect of booths with gems and minerals, beads, and fossil walrus tusk, all touted by Trader Rick as one of the greatest shows on earth. We immediately started scouting, our natural radar honing in on embellishments for our carvings. We held our fossil walrus carvings up to strands of semi-precious stone beads or balanced gemstones on their intricate detail to see how they'd look. This was dangerous territory. Bob took hold of the reins so I didn't get too crazy with my feeling that, 'An artist can never have too many tubes of paint or a beader too many beads'. While I was dancing between booths, looking at glorious strands of old African trade beads, he was looking at jewelry tools.

"Check out these glass and wood display cases." We'd done a New Year's Day show without a way to protect our pieces from sticky fingers. These were perfect and easily transportable. We bought three.

The booths were not only spread across acres and acres, but many different shows were all going on at once with RV accessories, crafts, household products, entertainment, food, gems, minerals, jewelry, and sculpture…phew! It was dizzying. There was camaraderie between young and old, hippies and blue-haired grandmothers, prospectors and cow folk coming together at this desert oasis. We camped in our van in a dusty parking lot filled with other people doing the same, got up in the morning and started the hunt all over again.

We came across Trader Rick's booth set up in front of his battered Airstream trailer. He gave us hints on where to find things and told us that Quartzsite was nothing compared to the shows in Tucson. He was going to fold his tent and caravan down there the following week.

We walked away with inspiration fluttering in our heads and spent two more nights in the parking lot, shopping by day until we dropped each evening, exhausted. Then destiny grabbed us by the hand and pushed us towards Tucson. Even though we'd brought our jewelry with us, we told ourselves, "We'll just go check it out for next year."

Once a year the city of Tucson morphs into the Gem and Mineral Show with gas stations renting out spaces to vendors and hotels turning their rooms into showrooms. A dirt lot becomes an African village, Persian rug salesmen hang their wares to undulate in the breeze so the patterns and colors beckon passersby to stop and inspect, and enormous crystals, six to ten feet tall, greet incredulous visitors. Tucson is Quartzsite on steroids. It's classy, huge, a twenty ring circus started in 1955 as a mineral club show at an elementary school that quickly grew, with more satellite shows cropping up every year.

Robert and Kathy from Heaven and Earth had a big showroom in The Pueblo Inn. They were thrilled to see us, and after hugs, Kathy said, "We have a table outside. We need someone to man it and direct people back here to us. If you want to do it, you can put some of your pieces out to sell."

"We're in business!" Bob agreed. And so started our twenty-four-year stint with the Tucson Gem and Mineral Show. We slept in our van in the parking lot, used friends' bathrooms to shower in and the hotel washing machine for our clothes. At the end of thirteen days we'd sold over four thousand dollars in necklaces and carvings, getting kudos for our work. "We're rich!" we high-fived, feeling we'd won the lottery or found that pot of gold at the end of the rainbow.

***

After two months of working diligently, my gynecologist convinced me to schedule a hysterectomy for fibroids, but I got scared and backed out. Instead, I decided to continue seeking alternative healers and therapies, hoping to avoid the knife. The thought of surgery terrified me, but the many stories I'd heard of women who'd healed themselves inspired hope. And that hope was echoed in Bali, known for its *balian*, or natural healers, some authentic, some quacks. We'd witnessed Bali's magic and experienced its nurturing environment, so it was natural for me to want to try alternatives before taking the allopathic route.

Years later, when Bob was diagnosed with Alzheimer's, our favorite balian, Tjokorda Rai, sadly admitted there was nothing he could do. I respected his honesty and genuine caring for Bob. Some things are incurable no matter the route taken. An authentic healer will acknowledge that.

***

Back in Bali, work and community kept us contentedly occupied with plenty of time for quiet meditations on the veranda. We continued to study Indonesian with Wayan Sidakarya until one day he told us, "I won a scholarship to do my master's degree at the University of Oregon. Do you know anyone who might want to buy my car?"

We looked at each other. Having seen so many motorbike accidents, I'd been wishing for steel around us. I just couldn't shake my nervousness when I was on the bike.

"Can we take it for a test drive?" Bob inquired. Off we went in the aging, paint peeling, dark green Toyota Land Cruiser. It was like driving a tank, but the price was right and we agreed to buy it. We named her Miss Daisy.

***

In July 1992 it was time for another visa run. I'd been using alternative therapies and trying to visualize the fibroids becoming smaller; I was sure they felt smaller when I pressed my hand along my abdomen. But Dr. Zovy, a gynecologist at Adventist Hospital in Penang, Malaysia had different news. She and the hospital came highly recommended, and when she told me the ultrasound showed my uterus was the size of a five-month pregnancy, I realized I'd lost the struggle. We scheduled surgery for ten days later.

I needed to organize a wire transfer since I didn't have health insurance. My mother and Helen both begged me over crackling phone lines not to have the operation in Malaysia, sending the fear of God through me, but I couldn't afford surgery in the States at a cost of five times more. They offered to lend me money if I'd do it in America, but my strong aversion to being in debt held me steady. At about five thousand dollars for the operation and recovery time in Malaysia, our savings account would be almost nil, but at least we could pay for it and be free.

While waiting, we took the train up to Bangkok. Our first stop was Harmonique to deliver an order and show Jacques and Boonma our newest designs. Our overflowing days camouflaged my fear until bedtime, when my demons came to taunt me.

Besides having an eye for style and outstanding objects, Jacques was also clairvoyant, a gift he'd had since he was a child. He'd become well-known for counseling and healing in Holland, but he'd left that life behind when he sold everything and set off to follow his own dreams. Yet sometimes the gift still demanded he surrender to it, and so he gave readings when he felt the pull. Often they were spontaneous.

When I told Jacques about my fears, his eyes glazed over, and with a different voice he said, "I see a caring woman who'll do her best surgery for you. You have a guardian spirit and there's light all around you. Try not to worry. Trust. This will open a new channel for you." I listened quietly. "You're strong, healthy, and a survivor, Susan. Try to relax." I breathed this in, more at ease, but not having a clue what the new channel would be.

The fear still dogged me, but when I could remember them, Jacques' words were an antidote. Back in Penang, I came down with flu two days before my pristine belly was to be forever altered. The surgery was postponed for two weeks. I felt so vulnerable and out of control, and yet I talked Bob into returning to Bali to take care of urgent concerns. Those two weeks without his support were excruciating. As soon as Bob left, all my fears rushed to the surface. Would I be awful during the pain of recovery, like a hurt animal lashing out at those there to help? I feared losing control and surrendering to my caregivers. I felt the real me lived behind a public persona, but I was no longer sure who was behind the mask. What if I didn't like what I saw? How could I cope with that? All my beliefs were on the line - my trust in life and my spiritual training. I was being stripped naked. Had I wasted twenty years meditating or would it guide me through this emotional jungle?

Handing a cassette tape to Dr. Zovy, I asked her to play my favorite music during the surgery. I asked that they not joke about me, but say affirmative statements, telling me how well I was doing and how I'd recover quickly, even though I was under anesthesia. These concepts were foreign to her, but she agreed. I also begged her not to take my ovaries if they were healthy.

This is the scariest thing I've ever had to do, I thought as I lay in bed the night before checking into the hospital. I watched my emotions rise and fall - fear, anxiety, elation, energy, and an attitude of I'll-whip-this. None of these feelings were stable. When I wasn't overwhelmed, I noticed a constant thread underlying every chaotic crumb of thought. Although emotions washed over me like waves on a beach, the sand was always there. Sometimes I couldn't see it for the water rushing in and out, but between waves there was clean, clear sand, anchored in the sunlight, connecting everything together. I tried to focus on that.

On the day of reckoning I was scared shitless, literally. I checked myself into the hospital alone, my voice and hands shaking, keeping an eye out for the nearest bathroom. I tried to quell the rising terror as I sat on the hospital bed weeping and knowing there was no way out. Bob wouldn't return until that evening, when I would be prepped for early morning surgery. At least he could sleep in the room with me so I wouldn't be alone.

The two and a half hour surgery took twice that, leaving Bob in near panic in the waiting room. Finally, a doctor came out. "It was a huge job - grandmothers and great-grandmothers of fibroids stuck to everything." The doctor went on to tell Bob that during the routine examination of my organs, they'd found a tumor inside my large intestine. They'd had to call in another specialist to remove about four inches of colon. We wouldn't know until the pathology came back if it was malignant. I'd lost a lot of blood and one ovary and they'd had to give me a transfusion.

The nurses didn't get me up for two days because of the severity of the ordeal. I counted the hours between pain injections and did exercises in bed, wiggling my toes, rotating my ankles, doing wrist and arm circles, and slowly rocking my pelvis. I knew movement was imperative for a speedy recovery. My first time up, I was so wobbly I could only go four steps, but with each subsequent effort I went further. By the next evening, I could walk the entire second floor, pushing my IV stand along with me. Ecstatic, I had a "Hello!" for everyone I passed.

With the help of caring staff, and by pushing myself to keep moving, I recovered so quickly that the doctors and nurses called me a model patient. Through it all, Bob was a model husband, always patiently there for me without being smothering. The first two days I couldn't stand to be touched except on my feet, so he massaged them or just held them and sent me healing energy. He got up several times a night to help me to the bathroom. It meant so much to me that he was there in the other bed, his gentle snoring soothing me when sleep was elusive.

Before we checked out, the pathology report came in. The tumor was from endometriosis and not malignant.

We moved into a guesthouse on the west coast of Penang for the month of recovery. The international guests included a Norwegian woman, a Saudi pilot and his Thai wife, a Libyan doctor, and a Taiwanese architect. None had been there less than three weeks. We fit right in, joining the sunset discussions out on the veranda.

Lui, the Chinese owner of the guesthouse, placed offerings on her Tao altar every day, including a glass of coffee, fruit, and incense, before she quietly recited her prayers. Her Hindu husband, on the other hand, powered around the guesthouse in fourth gear, shirtless in a white dhoti, wafting great plumes of incense smoke over Ganesha, Shiva, and a host of other Hindu images, and sending the guests scrambling for outside air.

Lui looked after me like I was a hurt bird. She cooked a special Chinese fish and herb soup believed to aid healing from surgery, boiled ginger footbaths and pampered me. Receiving didn't come easily to me, but I soaked it all in.

***

Fear wasn't ready to let go. We came home to Bali, our finances in a shambles, and faced eating into our only-in-case-of-dire-circumstances fund. Even with my mother gifting us food and accommodation for my recovery period, our doctor and hospital bills exceeded our bank account.

We plugged along producing carvings and jewelry and scouting handicrafts for Heaven and Earth and Savior Flair. When people realized we were in Bali to stay, we were accepted into a wider expat circle. There was also the start of a very special friendship, a friendship that would give me staunch support when Alzheimer's came along.

While I'd spent those two agonising pre-surgery weeks in Penang on my own, an American family had moved into the house next door to ours in Bali. Bob met Margie, Mitch, and their nine-year-old daughter, Ariana, when a house gecko (a lizard about eight inches long) got stuck on rat-glue paper we'd put out to get rid of vermin. Definitely not vermin, these shy, nocturnal creatures run up walls and across ceilings on velcro feet eating their fill of mosquitoes and other unwelcome insects. A rescue was needed.

"Can you help me with my gecko?" Bob asked Margie. Ariana volunteered to slip paper under each toe as Bob carefully released it with alcohol on a cotton swab. It was a long, tedious process.

"Bob, I can do this," said Ariana. "I know you're busy." So he left her to it.

As Bob got on with his errands, Ariana managed to free the gecko, but as soon as she had, it glommed onto her finger with its sharp teeth.

"Do lizards have rabies?" a worried Margie asked.

"No worries," said Bob, who put a little alcohol in the lizard's mouth to make him release his prey.

When I came back to Bali, Bob introduced me to our new neighbors. Both psychologists, they took time from their practices to see the world with their daughter during school holidays. Little did they know they too would fall in love with Bali and return year after year, making the island their second home. Our friendship grew with each summer's two month visit.

Again, time slipped by and our tourist visas required us to leave the country, so on December first we started a silent meditation retreat at Suan Mokh in Southern Thailand. We'd been to retreats there before, but this time we did two ten-day retreats, back to back. We both felt revived by these forays, and each retreat seemed to take on a different focus depending on where our minds were at the time. The theme this retreat was surrender and acceptance, tools we'd soon need.

***

Welcome to the USA! At customs, The Fish and Wildlife Department seized all of Bob's carvings while I got through with no problem. The customs agent claimed we needed a permit we'd never heard of to transport fossil walrus tusk across international borders. They couldn't give us any information on how we could obtain the permit and they fined us a thousand dollars on the spot to get our goods back. We were flabbergasted.

We talked with our suppliers and competitors. None had the permit or any inkling that it was necessary. After many phone calls and visits to the Fish and Wildlife office, they suddenly returned our check and told us they'd fine us through other channels. This never actually came to pass, but the fear of future seizures motivated us to continue our research. Eventually, we obtained the required CITES permit.

In spite of the glass cases we'd purchased at Quartzsite the previous year, four carvings were stolen at our annual New Year's Day show. We tried to convince ourselves that the thieves needed the pieces more than we did, but still it stung in spite of the many sales and compliments on our work.

But life's little ambushes weren't done with us yet. Nine days later, a friend called us. "Susan, Janet's house in Bali burned to the ground last night. Everything was lost. "

Normally we rented the house next door to Janet, but the owner had wanted it while we were away. We'd boxed everything up and stored it in Janet's loft, with the business valuables in a heavy wooden box. All our clothes, stones, beads, silver, fossil ivory, paintings, art supplies, tools, photos, books, and kitchenware had gone up in smoke. The cookie can storing our gemstones had melted around them, as did the plastic ice cube trays holding our beads. Most were unsalvageable.

A friend who sifted through the debris in search of anything useful found a charred bit of paper from our last meditation retreat. It read, 'Peace is found through non-attachment'. We had a good laugh over that.

Oddly, we took the news in stride. We'd finally surrendered to life leading us, seeing how little control we actually had. Then came the final coup. My remaining ovary had a rapidly growing tumor the size of a football on it and had to come out. We were in America with no health insurance and our emergency funds were gutted. With no other choice, we applied for county assistance, but the paperwork took so long that the operation was put off three times until the hospital was satisfied the state would pay.

In the meantime we went to Tucson to do the show again, only this time we not only manned the table for Heaven and Earth, we had a bigger display of our own work and bigger sales. People who'd bought the previous year came back. It was the start of a following. We used our profits to resupply after the fire loss, buying stones, beads, and fossil ivory.

While we were in Tucson, I had a dream in which I came across a very diseased man with an attendant. The man had a black oozing hole where one of his eyes should have been. He was bald except for black sores that sprouted a few hairs. He had a large opening in his abdomen and he was going through his intestines, cleaning them out with a crude, green metal appliance shaped like a dragon's head. He was obviously exhausted. The impatient attendant said, "As soon as you get this over with you can go to bed and have a little nap." I was so sorry for the man. I knew he spent most of his days doing this job.

This dream epitomized my fear of losing control of my life, of becoming a slave to debt, of facing the impending surgery, and of moving into middle age. Even though I was forty-seven, I clung to the image of being young and vibrant.

All the losses forced me to surrender or I'd go back into the dark pit. Gradually, something shifted, and while the fear didn't vanish, my whole attitude towards it changed. Sometimes I could surrender to the moment, to the fear itself or the fear of fear, and awareness backed it off. Sometimes the fear consumed me. Yet the fear became a teacher, as did the flirtations with surrender that would eventually become a serious union and bolster my foundation a decade later when we faced life with Alzheimer's.

Life was like a spiral, bringing me face to face with the same lessons over and over, but each time from a more heightened perspective. Even though we didn't know the nature of the tumor, I surrendered to not knowing. This time I wasn't afraid of the upcoming surgery in the way I'd been terrified about the first. Once again I healed quickly and learned the turmor was from endometriosis and not cancer.

After the surgery, Bob and I came to the difficult decision that we had to borrow money to keep our dream alive. With a friend's help and business acumen we made a plan, deciding to borrow more than we actually needed so we could jump-start our business. It wasn't easy to ask, but friends and family helped willingly, some not even wanting interest on their part of the loan. We set up payment schedules.

We were twenty thousand dollars in debt, but we felt loved. The debt was a mountain that kept us serious about Savoir Flair and disciplined in our work. Our footloose travelers' lifestyle was over.

Being stripped bare of so many things not only left us light and vulnerable, but also open to possibilities. We felt positive, almost giddy, full of gratitude for life with all its ups and downs. It felt as if we'd been taken by the hand and led through those experiences, and some day when we could look back, we'd see they led to something positive. That was where the trust came in. Through it all, Bob was my rock and stable place. Our love was growing stronger with each challenge.

Chapter Thirteen
Falling In Step With Alzheimer's

One could focus on the shards
The broken bits of events
Constantly shattered by the wheel of life
Or one can focus on the mending
Which can only happen in the OneTime
Now
Where nothing is
Ever
Other than whole

Between my surgeries, the fire, and using all our savings, we'd been stripped of our financial security in the early 90's. A decade later, Bob's mind is being stripped of memories, problem solving, and compassion.

It's raining and the electricity in Ubud is off again. My husband sits on the sofa with the phone book open on his lap. "Have you seen my wife?" he inquires when I come through the door. "I think she went to the gym, but I can't find the number."

I stare a beam of knowing into his eyes.

"Oh, not you! The other…" He trails off, getting a glimmer of how confused he is.

"I can't find my name in the phone book," he tells me. "What name does my sister go under?" He's desperately trying to make sense of his life. He doesn't remember that we live in Bali and aren't listed in the phone book. He doesn't remember that his sister lives in California. Or that she too has Alzheimer's.

After all these years I should be used to this, but still my heart races and my skin goes cold as I see Bob flailing, trying to get a grasp on reality. I force my emotions back so I won't cry and make him feel worse and more confused.

He closes the phone book and wanders into the bedroom. He takes his tee shirts off the shelves and folds them over and over again. Organizing calms him. I take a deep breath, push the sadness away, and sit on the veranda sofa to gather myself for afternoon work.

It's sunny and sprinkling rain all at once. Miraculously, this transports me to a pinpoint of peace where everything seems brighter, more vivid, sharper. I hear the sound of individual raindrops falling on leaves, the slap of Wayan's sandals as she breezes by with a tray of Balinese offerings, their incense wafting, and doves cooing behind the house. My thoughts stop. I'm suspended in timelessness. There's absolute joy for living, including all these hard and painful parts. I wish upon wish that I could share this, infuse Bob's heart with it.

It reminds of the feeling when the dragonfly suddenly appeared on Filicudi. I call it 'the special feeling' for lack of better words. My senses become hypersensitive to simple things like a single leaf curling to the ground or a cool breeze brushing my skin. I feel this is who I really am, and that I've forgotten it in the pain and responsibilities. Gratitude wells up. Grace has not forsaken me.

These intermittent revelations are part of the glue that keeps me adhered to the here and now. Without them, I'd surely crumble and float away. The other part that keeps me sane is my creativity. I've been painting for nearly a decade at a studio I rent just down the street from our house. I have a body of work, but no one has seen it except the people who the paintings are for.

I'll hear of someone in physical or emotional distress and sense that there's an image for them. I don't know how this image will help them, or even if it will, but it's so strong that I know I have to paint it. I sit and meditate, my mind emptying until the image comes. I try to stay true to what I see, or sometimes hear, as the painting evolves in my head. Occasionally, poetry accompanies it. I call these pieces 'Healing Maps'.

I paint them with dry pastels. When they're finished, I send a giclee print to the person that the image is for. People are often surprised by the particular image that comes to me for them, and frequently say their painting speaks to them deeply.

Once, a spider in a web appeared. I thought, *Oh no, I don't want a spider! They feel so threatening*. But I always try to stay as true to the image as possible. When I sent the spider painting to the woman it was for, a woman I'd only met once, she said, "I was unnerved to see the painting. I have a spider tatooed on my head that no one knows about. And I frequently feel wrapped up and encased in a web."

I also did one for Bob soon after his dementia became

apparent. It's a sparse piece done in colored pencil on ochre paper showing a treasure box slightly open and shafts of light radiating out. Bob didn't know what to say about it, but he keeps it on the wall where he can see it every day.

Since few of my friends have seen these artworks, I decide it's time to have a show. I haven't exhibited my paintings in twenty-five years.

At the opening, everyone greets Bob warmly, but he's clearly confused by the paintings and the gathering. He wanders over to a blond friend a little older than I and reaches to kiss her on the lips. Embarrassed by his strange advance, she turns her cheek. He takes her hand. She's wearing one of my mammoth tusk necklaces. When he whispers to her, "What a beautiful necklace you've made," it dawns on her that he thinks she's me.

"Your wife made this, Bob," she says, pointing me out across the room. The mask of confusion falls from his face as he releases her hand.

***

Bob was a frequent drinker when we met. He'd been bonding with his male friends over drinks ever since he first started sneaking into bars as a teenager. But he gave it up to please me, a non-drinker in those early years together. When he began meditation and we started traveling to Asia on a budget, alcohol slipped from his desires. Then slowly over time, we started to have an occasional cocktail with friends in Bali.

When we cared for my dying mother, we both drank a glass of wine with dinner every night as a way to relax and dull the intensity of the situation. In the early Alzheimer's years, Bob had no difficulty controlling his drinking. But an incident brought home to me that this has changed.

Margie and her husband, Mitch, Heiner, Bob and I are at Naughty Nuri's just outside Ubud, a place famous for its large, powerful martinis. Seated on benches around a communal, rough-hewn table, we're laughing, giggling, and having a great time. We raise our glasses to Heiner. "Here's to your new house!"

"Congratulations for taking the plunge!" I say.

"Here, here!" interjects Bob.

As soon as Mitch and Bob finish their drinks, they order another round. Margie and I usually split one, but this night we're especially happy for Heiner, and when we order dinner, we also order another round. Heiner, a beer drinker and lightweight, is happy with just one beer.

As the night progresses, Bob and Mitch seem to egg each other on to inebriation. Heiner insists, "I'm driving you all home."

He drops us off at our driveway. It's a full moon night and our door is about a hundred feet away along a narrow path atop a low embankment. I'm making my way in front of Bob when I hear a crash followed by laughter. I turn as he's hefting himself back onto the path, having veered off and fallen into a pile of garden leaves about four feet below. He thinks this is terribly amusing and doesn't seem hurt, but adrenaline shoots through my body and I sober up immediately. With a stern look, I thrust my hand out. "Bob, hold on to me. Walk slowly!"

We inch along, but almost at the entryway to our garden he topples over the other side of the path into a shallow pond. Again he comes up laughing, but this time covered in mud. My heart's pounding.

Once inside, I strip off his sodden clothes and lead him to the shower. He can barely stand up. I towel his clean body dry, but then face a dilemma. I need to get him some nightclothes, but I'm afraid to leave him. "Stand right here!" I command. "Don't move! I'll be right back."

I'm gone a few seconds when I hear a loud crash and moaning. Dashing back in, I see Bob sprawled out on the floor, semi-conscious, with a large egg forming on his head.

Now what the hell am I going to do? I run to the kitchen for ice for his head but I can't budge him and he can't stand on his own. I dash for the phone and call Heiner.

When he sees Bob laid out naked on the bathroom floor, he bursts out laughing, which gets me giggling at the absurdity of the scene. My stern expression melts. The egg, already responding to the ice, is shrinking. We get Bob up and into bed forgetting about nightclothes. He sleeps like the dead, but in the morning it's clear he's broken a few ribs. It's also clear that I'll have to monitor his drinking from now on.

I search the internet to read about Alzheimer's and alcohol use, but only find a caution that it could possibly interfere with medication and that it might exacerbate unsocial behavior. There's nothing more definitive.

At the same time that I'm realizing how much I need to keep

watch over Bob for his safety, I'm also learning where to let go of control when it isn't helpful.

We get home one evening, tired and grumpy after being away all day doing errands. I motion Bob to the couch. "Stay and relax, honey. I'll get us some snacks." I return with a ripe Camembert surrounded by thinly sliced pumpernickel and a small ceramic bowl of olives I'd marinated with garlic the week before. We both sigh into relaxation, gazing out at the garden as twilight descends and the garden lights come on.

"Honey, you take your shower first and I'll get dinner going. Then, I'll take mine," But when it's my turn to wash off the day's dust, Bob is busy turning off the outside lights and locking up the house. Our dining table is outside. So is the sofa where we usually relax until bedtime.

Fuming inside, I snap the lights back on and unlock the doors. I'm sitting on the sofa after our meal when he starts locking up again. "Bob, this feels awful. Let me relax out here!"

"I never do anything right!" He storms away.

"Can you just tell me why you want the light off so I can understand?" Of course, he can't explain. I consider this and wonder if it harkens back to growing up in the Depression and having to be careful of all expenditures, or perhaps during WWII when his coastal city was blacked out in case Japanese submarines attacked. Then I wonder if he's just bored or anxious. I realize I need to let this go for both our sakes and adapt to the situation.

*****

Our dear friend Mary, with whom we have Sunday brunch

whenever we're all in Bali, returns from a trip to England. "Susan, I have a gift for you. You'll hate it and love it. It's about Alzheimer's."

This book, *Contented Dementia* by Oliver James, becomes my guiding light over the next few months. Oliver's three basic commandments are: never ask questions, learn from the person with dementia, and always agree. So simple, and yet it's so hard to break old habits. Fortunately, there are strategies and details showing how to utilize the commandments.

I cry through the first section of the book because his understanding and compassion touch me so. I realize it makes sense to try to understand how the person with dementia perceives what is going on with them. The book shows how to give them a sense of security, making life easier for them and their caregivers.

The first commandment, not to ask questions, is a steep hurdle for me. A question like "Would you like a coffee?" requires a lot of recently stored information that a person with dementia simply doesn't have. The question sends them into a downward spiral of anxiety because they know they should be able to answer easily, but instead what might be going on in their mind is a set of other questions such as: What time is it? Is it too late to have coffee? Have I had coffee today? This inner questioning often leads them astray until they don't even remember the original question. Yet there's someone looking at them, waiting for an answer while they fruitlessly sift through whatever thoughts are coming. Panic arises, but they try not to show it.

I begin to lead with statements like, "I feel like a cup of coffee," while looking directly into Bob's eyes. This usually prompts him to say, "I'll have one too." Or I yawn and say, "It's time for me to go to bed." He takes the cue and agrees he's tired too.

Then I work with the second commandment – to learn from Bob. I make a list of things Bob used to talk about that are part of his distant history, such as family outings to a nudist camp, running on the beach as a toddler, spending summers on Catalina Island, or how his mother got him to like raw veggies. I grow the list to twelve topics. The book is making welcome changes to my relationship with Bob. Using a verbal game that Oliver suggests, we start to have dinner conversations again, and while they're staged by me, at least Bob is talking.

I toss out a morsel. "This dinner is really delicious, Bob." He nods and keeps eating. "You've been lucky to have such good cooks in your life, like your Mom, Clare and me."

His eyes light up. I can see his mind is searching, "My mom used to take raw peas and put them in an old cheese jar with mayonnaise. I'd toddle off eating them with my fingers." He takes a bite of dinner.

I egg him on with another morsel. "I love peas."

He takes the bait. "Sometimes she'd put in carrot or celery sticks. She got me to appreciate vegetables early on."

Bob is smiling, feeling good about himself, and I'm delighted to not be sitting in silence. The conversation moves from his mother, to times at the nudist camp, to being married to Clare. I'm new to these techniques, but I love a challenge and jump in full force to change how I behave with Bob. What's so satisfying is when I find the right topic, he lights up and talks and all I have to do is add a few head nods or "Uh huhs," or "You were really lucky," to corroborate what he's saying.

Oliver validates something I've always felt – Bob, my soulmate, is still in there. He has a terminal disease that erases his mind's ability to store new information, but if I give him a sense of security and confidence, more of him will come out. This means I have to suspend what I think of as common sense and rational thinking, and enter his world. I also have to learn the third commandment: to always agree with him by using the art of redirection and actual fibbing.

If Bob says it's hot when it's cold, I just agree. If he says he wants to go for a ride, I say, "What a good idea! We can go in about half an hour." Of course, he'll have forgotten it by then.

The book comes at the right time as so much of the help I've received on this journey has. I marvel at how lucky I've been over the years with people, information, or morsels of inspiration appearing just when I've needed them. A basic trust in life has slowly replaced the old ever-present fear. This was validated and cemented into place by a wise, elderly Indian sage.

Chapter Fourteen
Touched by Angels

Grace tapped me gently on the shoulder
A touch so light it almost went unnoticed
I turned to see who was there
And saw my Self reflected in a thousand mirrors
Each face different
Each face the same

Time disappeared in quicksand moments on the Island of the
Gods, which we now called home. With our recent losses
and the urgent need to pay back our loans, I knuckled under
designing jewelry and sculpture. Our debt weighed heavily on
our sense of freedom.

Bob roughed out material and interfaced with the carvers in
their village, keeping an eye on quality and rejecting anything
not up to our standards. We were a good team and it felt like we
were grabbing hold of life. In survival mode, working seven
days a week, there was little time for art, poetry or friends.

Margie pursued me persistently, not giving up on our
fledgling friendship. We laugh now at how rude I was, feeling
the need to work seven days a week. Since phones were rare,
she'd show up unannounced at the house we'd recently moved

to, out in the ricefields, "I have to work!" I'd growl at her, barely looking up after she'd walked half an hour in the humid heat.

I'm so grateful she hung in there. Our deep, lasting friendship has seen us both through difficult times. Even years later when I was a crazed caregiver, she never wavered. She learned to endure Bob's hostility as anger accompanied him through the haze of Alzheimer's. He'd shout, "I don't need two wives!" and stomp off when Margie tried to help him with a difficult task

Not happy out of town in the rice paddies, we rented two tourist rooms at Sanjiwani, a home stay on the edge of Ubud. One room became Bob's workshop and the other our bedroom. The communal space joining them morphed into a living room/ studio/office with a kitchen at the far end. Victoria, a woman I'd met at Sania House in 1988, moved into the room across from us. She was looking for an alternative place to the States to live and earn a living. A loosely woven family emerged between the three of us and the owners of the place.

It was still a time of change. Geoff left Gill for a younger woman in Paris, but Gill kept the Bali house and the life they'd built with their Balinese family and expat friends, who all rallied around her in support. After a year of grief she smashed out of it and took Bali by storm photographing and writing about her passion – the trance ceremonies of this mystical culture.

At Sanjiwani Bob and I worked ferociously. Laughter took a vacation as we put what money we had into stock for the next Tucson show, eating as cheaply as we could and cutting costs whenever possible. The possibility of earning enough in Tuscon to pay our obligations and keep our dignity with family and friends who believed in us kept us moving forward.

Despite the mounting pressure, creativity still managed to push through. During one of our evening meditations I had a vision of a new logo and name for our business. I saw a globe of the world with turquoise landmasses hanging from a thread on sand-colored paper with dark plum lettering. It not only reflected our collection of beads from all over the world strung into necklaces, but also our carving material from Alaska transported to Bali. And it reflected our life philosophy. Savoir Flair transformed into 'World on a String'.

In spite of the hardships we'd endured, we felt that living in Bali we had 'the world on a string, sittin' on a rainbow,' as the song says. We'd had a tsunami of challenges, but when the waters receded, there we were in paradise feeling the magic and working in a manner that fed our souls and tickled our creativity. And we knew how lucky we were to have Tucson only once a year as the major outlet for our work.

***

"I can sell this stuff!" exclaimed a scruffy man in ripped jeans and matching jacket. He had a mop of frizzy hair sticking out from under a denim cap. He'd bought from us the previous year, selecting our best Buddha and Kuan Yin sculptures, and hadn't quibbled about the price. Now here he was again at our Tucson show, looking through our cases and getting excited. His eyes darted from one piece to another.

"I'll take all those." He pointed at a three-tiered glass case, "And that one, and the one over there. Hell! I'll take them all!"

I lifted up the table skirt hiding our extra stock. "How about these?" I asked.

"Yes, throw those in too."

"What about our friend Mauro's work? These fabulous gold and gemstone pendants?" Mauro shared our Tucson booth, but was off for a break.

"Hmmm." The scruffy man looked over the work. "Yes, I'll take all of those."

My ears were buzzing and my heart pounding. This was too good to be true. I had to remind myself to breathe. The first nine days of the show had been alright, but not what we'd hoped for.

"In fact," he interrupted my mental mutterings, "I'll even take your display cases. Wrap them well so they don't break."

"I have a nice pair of dirty socks here," I quipped.

He laughed. "Write it all up and have it inventoried and packed by Saturday. There'll be a truck to pick everything up." And with that he left our booth and left us trying to re-hinge our jaws.

"Was he serious?" Bob looked like a stunned mullet. This was an artist's dream come true. But there were four show days left and he'd asked us to stop selling and start packing. No money had changed hands. All we had was his promise and the hope of ending our debt worries.

The din grew louder as Gregory Spellman made his way through the show. Sometimes he purchased whole booths, sometimes just a few pieces; some displays he walked right by, leaving a trail of jubilance and disappointment as he moved down the aisles. As word spread, people thronged him, vying for his attention. By the end of the day he'd agreed to spend more than two million dollars, mostly without a penny in deposit.

When we walked into the show the next morning after a sleepless night, Lee, whose booth had also been sold in its entirety, had a rope strung across his entrance with a sign, 'Closed, Gone Fishin'. He'd done a little research and learned that Gregory had made a fortune with alternative health products. He'd sold some stocks that were not 'politically correct' and had a vision to reinvest in art. He may have looked like a hippy, but beneath the garb was a savvy businessman. We started inventorying and packing.

On Saturday the truck arrived as promised. I waited nervously, shifting from one foot to the other while his ragtag staff organized themselves. I handed over our whole inventory, our display, our entire business and our future, and in return received a check for $39,000. I studied it in disbelief. Would it clear? There was nothing to do but trust.

We felt touched by Grace. This man changed our lives with an eight by three-inch piece of paper, a few ink strokes, and a completely illegible signature. He gave us enough to pay off our remaining loans and to invest in our business, to take risks with higher quality stones and use gold more often instead of only silver. We had wriggle room to make outrageous or expensive pieces that might not sell right away. He gave me a chance to design for art's sake instead of designing only what I thought would turn over quickly. I will always feel grateful to the man in the tattered jeans.

***

The years tumbled one into another. Our business grew to twenty-five employees, mostly carvers, and while it wasn't a wild success, it was supporting us all. A couple of times a year, visa runs gave Bob and I the opportunity to see more of South-East Asia, deepening our love for this part of the world and for each other with each new exploration.

Our friends called us 'SusanandBob', pronounced as one word, and said we were joined at the hip. I loved our connection and companionship, but still sought alone time to maintain my inner balance. Bob never pressed me on this, easily giving me the freedom and support I needed.

Tom, our old friend from the early days, suffered a stroke while in Bali and spent a night and part of a day unable to move until he was found by staff at his guesthouse. His daughter, Linda, air evacuated him home to Australia. We continued to write when he recovered that ability, but he wasn't able to return to Bali. Then the letters stopped. We missed Tom and his wild stories and our discussions about art and the creative process.

Then in 1995 the dreaded 'C' word entered our world. Bob was diagnosed with bladder cancer at Bangkok's Adventist Hospital. We were still stunned by the diagnosis as he was wheeled into surgery to remove a stage two tumor, but relieved when we learned that this is a fairly easy cancer to treat. It would take six weeks of BCG treatment – a bacterial drug also used to prevent tuberculosis.

The idea of being away from Bali for six weeks was too depressing. We talked the doctor into teaching us how to administer the treatment ourselves at home. It required inserting a catheter through the penis into the bladder and then mixing the BCG with a saline solution and injecting the mixture into the catheter, keeping everything as sterile as possible. The process seemed daunting. Bob had to hold this liquid in for an hour, a feat he was rarely able to do. When we returned to Bangkok eight weeks later, we found the treatment had worked. He was given the all clear, but would need to be monitored every six months for the next five years.

Twelve months later, on the second monitoring, the cancer was back. Bob had surgery to remove the new tumor, and again we went home armed with catheter, BCG vials, and saline. Like the year before, I was a ball of nerves doing this procedure, fearing I'd accidently introduce infection into him. I was also scared that I'd lose my soulmate to this disease. It had come back in spite of doing everything we were supposed to do, including eating a mostly macrobiotic, alkaline diet with little refined sugar.

Because of the recurrence, I was more jumpy and tense than the first time, worrying someone would interrupt us in the middle of the process, so Margie volunteered to stand guard at our door, barring anyone who came calling while we did the weekly treatment. This time it was a success and Bob remained cancer free for the rest of his life.

***

In the late 90's I lost my parents. Mom had already been

diagnosed with metastasized cancer when my father passed away from prostate cancer. My sister, Joan, and Bob and I cared for her at her home during her last three months, showering her with attention, compassion, and humor. She was an easy, appreciative patient and we four had a lot of laughs in those precious few months. She looked at us one day and said, "I never realized I was so loved." The love was palpable, and what a joy it was to give back for the gift of life she gave Joan and me.

For years, our mother had asked us to put our initials on the bottoms of objects in the house that we would want when she 'went to her reward', as she referred to death. We'd laughed it off, but now she insisted we go through her closet and jewelry box, choosing what we each wanted.

It was a highly emotional afternoon. There were no squabbles between Joan and I; all we wanted was our mother. In the choosing, the three Balinese sculptures that had inspired me as a child became mine while Joan chose delicate jade carvings. But the real inheritance was the bond cemented between us in these months of care-giving.

One afternoon Mom announced, "I'm ready to go, and I've decided it'll be tonight. Let's have a farewell party." Bob volunteered to do the grocery shopping, getting a bottle of her favorite Gewürztraminer. We propped her up in bed and tied colorful ribbons in her hair. In a gay mood, she wrapped a silk scarf around her shoulders. Dad's ashes were moved to the dresser next to her and drinks were poured. We reminisced, cracking jokes whenever we could, and getting downright silly.

She had a tiny sip of her wine while we downed ours, trying to keep the tears away.

It was a slice of gaiety, a celebration of life, even though she was unable to eat more than a smidgen of the fare we'd prepared. We knew she was in a bad way when she refused her favorite smoked salmon. She lasted less than an hour before she was too tired to go on and asked us to put her to bed.

By then she could no longer put her dentures in or get to the bathroom on her own. Bob lifted her carefully onto a portable bedside toilet and left her to her business. Joan or I went in to clean up before Bob returned to put her back in bed. This once elegant, dignified woman looked so small and fragile in his muscular arms. None of the three of us slept well that night, fearing her loss yet wanting her to be free of pain.

The next morning the air was red with swear words blasting from the bedroom. Disgusted and disheartened, Mom woke up to a new day. She lasted a few agonizing weeks longer, losing more and more of her dignity as she slipped into helplessness. Finally, after four days in a coma, her wish was granted.

Our love for this woman made it a privilege to be there for her. It was a highlight of both Joan's and my life, and brought us closer than we ever imagined. It also showed me a deeper side of Bob and his capacity for compassion and caring. He was our support team, running to the store at a moment's notice, helping with chores, cracking jokes, and showing a deep love for our mother in everything he did.

***

Mom's death left a void in my spirit and a revived hunger

to know Truth. At the suggestion of a friend, I started reading books on Advaita, a philosophy from India that says: Events happen, deeds are done, but there is no individual doer thereof. In other words, nothing is personal – we are actors in a play that is directed by God, Consciousness or Source and is acted by God, Consciousness or Source. All our emotions, feelings, suffering, joy, pain and pleasure are expressions of the Source of All.

If one really lived this, it would be the end of guilt, the end of hatred and malice, the end of suffering in the mind. All that would be left is inner peace. This way of thinking spoke to me on a deep level. The void filled with Advaita.

In 2000 Bob met Don, a traveler who'd just come from India where he'd been seeing a sage called Ramesh Balsekar, who espoused Advaita. Don was glowing. Bob said to me, "We have to meet this sage. I want some of what Don has!" We made vague plans to go, but in the end they didn't gell.

The next year Bob ran into Don again and he was glowing even more. He told us Ramesh was authentic, but old, and people were having dreams that he would die soon. Bob said, "We really have to go to India. Let's make a plan now!" That plan put us in Bangkok, getting our Indian visas, on September 11, 2001.

The news of what was happening in the States had us in shock and turmoil. It seemed the world would come to an end. We didn't know what to do. Should we continue on to India? In the end we agreed that if the world was in serious danger, what better place to be than sitting with an enlightened master?

We were late that first morning, having lost our way trying to find Ramesh's house in southern Mumbai. His sitting room was already jammed with over twenty visitors, so we were directed to a couch outside, but within earshot, and from where we could catch glimpses of him from the doorway. Those images stayed with me throughout the day, often bringing me to tears. My heart felt so open and vulnerable, leaving me confused as to why this was happening. I'd only glimpsed the man.

The next morning about a dozen of us gathered on the sidewalk across the street from where Ramesh lived. Murti, the man in charge, asked us to wait for his signal before we ascended the five flights of well-worn stairs to Ramesh's top floor apartment. Tension and anticipation grew as we waited. Murti asked Bob if he wanted to have a discussion with Ramesh, but Bob declined, not knowing what to say. I thought, *I've come all this way – I'm going to use this time wisely,* not knowing they called the chair I would be directed to 'the hot seat'. Finally, Murti told us it was time to go up.

I was nervous, folding and unfolding my hankerchief as we waited for the old sage to appear. He came down the hall from his bedroom, clicking his dentures in place and stopping in front of photos of his teachers. He raised his pressed together hands to them in *namaste*, the Hindu greeting that means, 'The divine in me acknowledges the divine in you'. He entered the sitting room namasteing to the twenty-two of us crammed in there, and sat down in front of the gathering and right in front of me.

He asked me my name, what part of the world I was from

and what I did for a living. Then he asked why I was there. I said I wanted to know Truth.

"Tell me, Susan, what have you done up to now to know this Truth?"

I told him about my experience with the pelicans when I was sixteen and how that loss of myself to the moment began my spritual quest. Tears welled up and spilled over, and I said, "That experience is what is happening right now with you. And I don't know why I'm crying." It felt as if the rest of the room had disappeared, and only Ramesh and I were present.

He asked me if I'd read any of his books. I told him which ones, and that I'd printed thirteen pages from his website and had almost read the print off of them. "Every time I read these concepts, they go in deeper." It was hard to speak - tears kept getting in the way.

Ramesh said, "Don't worry about the emotions."

I told him I'd been meditating for nearly thirty years, but recently I'd felt it was time to stop. Every day, all day, had become a meditation, so sitting just dropped off.

"In other words, meditation happened and meditation unhappened?"

"Even seeking unhappened. And that feels strange since I've been a seeker since I was sixteen. Now, I just want to be with what is. And even when it's uncomfortable, there's peace behind it."

Ramesh asked me about finding his website and what happened. "When I saw your photo, I knew we absolutely had to come and meet you. With all the reading and meditation I've done, I've never found a teacher. In fact, I'm not looking for a teacher now."

"Well, has the teacher found you?" Ramesh was a little emotional too.

"So, now, is there something you want from me, Susan?"

"No, just to be here."

Ramesh began his discourse, explaining that consciousness is all there is. There are no individual doers. "And when the idea 'thy will be done' goes deep into your heart, you are left with peace." Nothing in the outer world changes, just your attitude to it.

That meeting was another life changer.

After a few years of visiting Ramesh and taking his teachings in, I realized that I was no longer run by fear. Instead, fear had transformed itself into my ally and guide. All I was required to do was observe its antics. I saw how it functioned as a response to something brushing up against my senses or to a thought. It wasn't personal. It was just how the mind works.

Instead of being plowed under when fear stampeded, I learned to step aside and watch it go by. Occasionally, though, almost as a reminder to stay vigilant, it would sneak up from behind. But it could no longer fool me. When I looked back, I wondered, *Who was that Susan who was sitting on thorns so much of her life?*

Bob reacted to this unconscious change in me in a manner I would never have expected. Mr. Mellow, who'd rarely worried about the future, suddenly started. It was as though one of us had to take on the role of Nervous Nelly for our bond to be stable. Perhaps this was an early glimmer of dementia taking hold.

Chapter Fifteen
Alz World - Early Years

Alzheimer's is a disease of silent loss
It creeps up
Stealing the night
Right from under your nose

My mother placed steaming cappuccinos and my favorite dark chocolate dipped shortbread cookies on a plate between us. We were sitting at her kitchen table on a cool spring day in 1985 overlooking the pine-studded foothills of Nevada City, California.

I cleared my throat a few times too many. "Is there something you want to talk about?" she asked.

"You know how much Bob and I are in love, right? And you know what a great guy he is." I paused, searching for the right words. My mother had been through two marriages, an annulment and a divorce with me. "Well, we've decided to get married next year."

She dunked her cookie into the hot coffee, chewing thoughtfully. "Susan, you're fifteen years younger than Bob. I know he's a good man. And I know he loves you a lot." She hesitated, until her eyes met mine. "But try to imagine when you're my age, seventy-three. You'll most probably be a widow. Or caring for a frail old man."

"Look at your father and me. We never thought we'd get this old." Dad had always maintained the outside of the house, but now, with his heart problems, Mom was having to roll the cans for weekly garbage pick-up down their steep driveway to the street. More than once she thought their weight would run away with her. And having to push the empty cans up the drive was not much easier. "I don't say this because I don't want you to be happy," she went on. But I don't want to see you hurt either."

Although I knew she only wanted to protect me, I was disappointed. I'd wanted her to be happy for me, for the love Bob and I shared. I took a deep breath. "I'd rather have some fantastic years of deep love and joy than try to be safe, Mom. I'll take what comes along with that."

And that's how I've lived my life. Being an artist leads to an uncertain future, living in Indonesia doesn't give much security, and traveling to third world countries as a backpacker is risky. Safety is obviously not what I think about. Love has always been my priority.

***

After my brush with death in 2000, when I had to have emergency surgery in Bali for a strangulated intestine, it became obvious to our friends that something was wrong with Bob. I was in denial, but when I look back now I see there were signs I didn't see then. The stories he'd tell about our adventures had me wondering who he'd traveled with because I sure didn't have the same experiences. This made me doubt my own memory.

Bob had always been forgetful with his keys, glasses and wallet; he'd discovered he'd forgotten his driver's license on our first date when we were pulled over by a policeman. But gradually this increased, as did his confusion when he tried to find objects. His short-term memory was decreasing. I told myself these could just be signs of normal aging, and being absent-minded was just part of who he was.

But Bob was so concerned about these lapses we had him tested on our annual return to the States that year. For five hundred dollars we were told there was nothing wrong and the tester only hoped he'd be in as good mental shape when he reached Bob's age. This wrong information nailed my denial to the ground.

In an aside, the tester mentioned there was a slight possibility Bob might have Mild Cognitive Impairment. For another five hundred they could do further testing to see if that was the case. We opted not to continue. We had the news we so wanted to hear: *Bob was normal*.

Yet over the next year or two, my sweet husband transformed, at times, into a misogynist, taking on a new, biting attitude towards me. He'd parry with sarcastic jabs tossed out in front of friends, like the time we were having dinner with our next-door neighbors, Jean and William. While catching up on each other's news, Bob told them about a man we'd met in the States. "Victoria's man, Sam, introduced us to a possible good business connection."

"No, it was Simon," I corrected, "and Ginia introduced us."

Bob glared at me and continued, "So this Simon has several galleries in LA."

"New York," I said meekly, not wanting to rock the boat but feeling this needed to be accurate.

He bellowed, "Can't I say anything without you interrupting me! I can talk and think on my own, you know! You're such a control freak!"

I apologized and let him continue telling the story with all its misinformation, embarrassed at times that he was so far off the mark.

Later, Jean pulled me aside and said, "Susan, I don't know how you take Bob talking to you like that."

"I barely notice it, Jean. It goes right over my head." I pondered this a minute and then said, "I know he loves me." I was covering for him and I didn't even realize it.

But other friends noticed that Bob was becoming short with them, irritated over seemingly benign actions or comments. Margie went away in tears a few times after Bob berated her for talking too much or being over-enthusiastic. At first, I think we all believed he had control over his actions and that he was simply becoming a grumpy old man.

Yet with more and more observations from friends, I began to notice his jabs. I started to take it personally. I'd stop Bob and say, "Please don't talk to me that way." He'd look perplexed, not really understanding what I was talking about. He nicknamed me Gloria or called me Nervous Nelly, with sarcasm rather than humor in his voice.

If he perceived I was watching him, even in a loving way, he'd say, "Stop trying to manage my every move! You don't need to watch me. I've lived seventy years taking care of myself!" This wasn't the open, caring Bob I'd married.

Bob started getting annoyed with our staff as well. He was becoming increasingly intolerant and distrustful, and even worse, disrespectful. He knew something was terribly wrong but he couldn't do anything about his actions. And he was still sharp enough to remember that this disease was in his family. He felt helpless and depressed and talked about ending his life, a topic that came up whenever he thought he was getting forgetful, which was happening more frequently.

Finally, we consulted a doctor in Bangkok who ordered an MRI to rule out tumors and blood clots, which can cause symptoms similar to Alzheimer's. Bob was eager to find out what was going on, but at the same time afraid to know.

Looking at the results the doctor said, "I hope my brain will be in such good shape when I'm Bob's age." He told us the MRI showed a normal brain for a seventy-one year old man. Wrong information part two and more false hope. We didn't know then that in the early stages of Alzheimer's the MRI may be normal, not yet showing the atrophy that typically comes later.

But on our trip to the States in 2004 it was no longer possible to ignore reality. We were directed to a well-respected psychiatrist who, after taking Bob's history, prescribed Aricept, an acetylcholinesterase inhibitor. Acetylcholine is a neurotransmitter in the brain that is necessary for memory and cognition. In Alzheimer's disease it gets broken down. Aricept slows down the process in some patients.

The psychiatrist told us, "Given Bob's history and symptoms, he probably has Alzheimer's. There's no set way to diagnose the disease. It's a matter of deduction. We eliminate other causes to conclude the person has AD." I clung to the words, "he probably has Alzheimer's" with 'probably' in capital letters.

There's no cure for Alzheimer's, but Aricept and other, newer drugs are used to slow down the progression of symptoms to give a better quality of life. Unfortunately, this doctor was another professional who did us a disservice by giving us wrong advice because, like many doctors who aren't specialists in the disease, he really knew little about it. He told Bob what I'd been suspecting. "You just don't try hard enough to remember. You're leaving things to Susan. She's become your memory. And like any muscle, if you don't use it, you lose it." I was secretly cheering inside. I was so sure we could fight this thing, but I knew I couldn't do it without Bob's help. Later, I discovered it's common for caregivers of those with early stage Alzheimer's to try to get the person to rejoin them in their world as they see them slipping away. Our friends validated this idea and encouraged Bob to try harder. But the meeting with the doctor had left Bob feeling he was a failure and sent him further into depression. "I'm useless,' he told me. "I'm just making your life difficult. I think I should do us both a favor and do myself in."

With a Pollyanna outlook, I did what I could to lift Bob's spirits. We signed him up for further Indonesian language lessons in Ubud, since he hadn't kept up with his lessons from the early years. Learning a language is a good way to exercise the gray cells. We picked out crossword puzzle books and dictionaries for further mind exercises, even though Bob had never had any interest in crosswords and was always a bad speller. I was grasping at straws. The books sat on the shelf unopened. He did read *Improving Your Memory for Dummies* and *The Complete Idiot's Guide to Improving Your Memory.* He seemed to get a lot out of these, often looking up to read me a passage. But the book he spent the most time with, underlining and circling pertinent points, was *Brain Longevity* by Dharma Singh Lhalsa, MD. On page twenty-one he circled, in black ink, 'There's No Such Thing as a Hopeless Case'.

But hopeless or not, Bob couldn't remember anything from these books for long. This happened with novels as well as newspaper and magazine articles. Eventually, he'd pick them up and open them anywhere just to have something to do. It was the reading that mattered, not getting anything out of the words.

I mistakenly thought Bob wasn't trying hard enough to remember, that he was somehow being lazy. I thought when he was taking language lessons that he just needed to study and practice more.

One of the hardest concepts for families and friends to understand and accept is that a person with Alzheimer's doesn't actually forget new memories. Those events are never stored to begin with. It's as though their RAM is full, so new experiences or knowledge never get sent to the hard drive for later retrieval. And they can't help this.

What makes this particularly difficult to accept is that, in the early years, people with Alzheimer's function normally most of the time. But there are holes in their reality where they act differently to what the people around them are used to, and this completely throws us off our footing. We think they can control these 'holes' and behave as they used to. We try to get them to rejoin us in our reality. But this isn't possible. Until we accept this and meet them in their world, we suffer tremendously.

***

Without the foundation of Advaita, I could have easily been consumed by future-tripping anxiety when Bob was diagnosed with Alzheimer's, but I wasn't. I took it as a challenge. I was determined I wouldn't be victim to it and I didn't spend much time thinking about what would come to pass.

Over the years I'd learned through Ramesh, retreats, books and my own experience that the greatest healer is awareness. The mere observation of what is going on in the mind - without changing it, wanting to change it, or resisting it - causes change to happen. But you can't orchestrate that change. It happens naturally and this requires trust – trust in life. And I'd learned that awareness brings acceptance on it's heels, acceptance of what is, in the moment. Both of these attributes helped me as a caregiver. I sensed that all the soul-searching at retreats, the year with Helen and Lisa, all the inner angst, fear, and finally, acceptance, had prepared me for this part of our life together. These tools were my arsenal; they were to get us through the first eight years of the disease with relatively few meltdowns.

Friends marveled at how I was able to hold everything together, take care of Bob, and at the same time, work to support our loyal team of workers. When people queried, "What'll you do when he wanders at night, can't communicate, is incontinent?" I told them I'd jump off that bridge when I came to it, usurping one of Gill's favorite twisted metaphors. Although I suspected these years of stress were gathering ammunition behind my back, waiting for an ambush, I vowed to stay strong. "I can do this, I can do this, I can do this," I told myself.

We saw Ramesh every year until he passed away in 2009. His teachings solidified the foundation I needed to deal with Alzheimer's and to be as good a caregiver as I could be. In the early years of Alzheimer's, our visits to the old sage gave Bob solace. He felt Ramesh accepted him for who he truly was beyond the disease.

***

In the fall of 2004, with Bob having been on Aricept for nine months, we traveled to Sri Lanka and southern India for five weeks. Bob had always been the brawn, carrying our luggage, and also watching out for me to make sure I was safe. He'd put himself in danger before he'd let me face it. But Alzheimer's was eroding the gallant man.

One day, getting into the car with our driver, Bob said in a serious tone, "Susan, you ride up front so if anything happens I'll be OK in the back." My heart sank. The fact that my White Knight was no longer watching out for me sank deeper into my psyche when we had to cross chaotic Asian streets. Pre-Alz, Bob would take my hand while he assessed the situation. When he saw a safe gap, he'd give me a tug and we'd run across together. In Sri Lanka, I was off his radar. I had to fend for myself, with him fuming on the other side because I didn't run when he did. We were back full circle to our first trip to Asia before we'd worked out how to cross the streets together.

Always gregarious and outgoing, Bob had never been afraid to talk to strangers, but with Alzheimer's he knew no limits. He could no longer sense when it wasn't a good idea to interrupt or approach strangers. He'd pass a table and start talking, usually sure he already knew the people, although I knew we'd never met them. Or he'd talk to other customers in stores or folks on the street in a way that made them uncomfortable, or at least made me uncomfortable. I imagined having a disclaimer card: *My husband has Alzheimer's and can't help his behavior.*

Mornings in Sri Lanka often ended in panic as we packed to travel to a new location. I kept all the important papers, such as air tickets and passports, credit cards and contacts, but Bob had pocket money. I'd see him searching his pockets or going through books in a cloud of anxiety, tearing bedding apart, or pulling drawers out to look under and behind them.

"What's wrong, Honey?"

"I can't find my money. I put it somewhere safe last night. But I can't remember where."

We'd hired a car for ten days to take us to many of the World Heritage Sites on the island. Harry, our driver, was soon impatient having to delay morning departures. We'd pull Bob's bag out of the trunk and go through it looking for the cash, which usually turned out to be in the pocket of pants he'd worn the day before. Harry also became increasingly impatient with Bob's repeated questioning, "What's on the schedule for today?" "Where are we?" or "When do we eat?" The questions cycled over and over. The tension built until we were happy to be on our own again a week later.

My need for alone time in the early mornings finally overcame me. Having time to wander at my own pace and photograph saved my sanity. I didn't need more than an hour and a half to be revived and ready to go back to Alz World, so I continued a technique I'd been using for a couple of years - leaving notes for Bob taped to the door or bathroom mirror or both. 'I've gone for a walk and will return at 8:30 so we can have breakfast together. Please do not leave the hotel!' This ploy continued to be useful until a year later, when I lost Bob in Laos.

That 2004 trip to Sri Lanka brought home just how serious the situation had become. Having Harry, a complete stranger, reflect back to me how compromised Bob's memory was, startled me out of denial.

In Bali, Bob seemed more normal. He could still drive and do errands without me, providing he had a list, and he could still do his work as long as he had written instructions and could come to me to confer. But out in the world I'd seen his reality cracking.

In 2005 we took a trip with our good friend, Heiner, to Luang Prabang, a small, beautifully preserved city, which was once the capital of Laos. Heiner had another close friend with Alzheimer's, so he was supportive and sympathetic. That trip was a turning point.

I'd gone out for my morning alone time leaving the usual note taped to the door: 'I am out for a walk and will be back at

8:30 am. Please don't leave the hotel.' As an extra precaution, I put the hotel's business card in Bob's belly pack. But when I returned with fresh-baked croissants to dunk in the sweet Lao coffee provided in the hotel's garden, our room was empty. The hotel's card lay on the desk along with assorted items my husband deemed not needed for the day.

Heiner hadn't seen Bob and the staff simply said, "He go out." Heiner and I waited, sipping our coffee, munching croissants, and trying not to worry. But after ninety minutes, anxiety shook us into submission.

We decided the best course of action was to rent bicycles and search in different directions. We bargained for the bikes and paid a deposit, but just as we were ready to take off, Bob came hurrying towards us, fear and relief alternating on his face.

"Where have you been!" he demanded, trying to cover his tracks. I was so relieved to see him I didn't get angry that he'd forgotten my instructions. I didn't even get angry with myself for not seeing that what had worked for a couple of years was no longer viable. Notes taped to doors were useless. Bob had reached the stage where he couldn't be left alone.

A few evenings later we were at Luang Prabang's famous night market, a kaleidoscope of Hill Tribe costumes and handicrafts. Bob and I were looking at handbags assembled with bits of old weavings and antique glass beads. Suddenly, he needed to find a bathroom. To avoid an accident we had to act quickly. Incontinence, a common symptom and consequence of Alzheimer's, develops as the mind/body communication becomes damaged. Physical signals we take for granted are not read by the mind until it's almost too late. Eventually, the signal can't be read at all, and in late stage Alzheimer's total incontinence becomes the daily norm.

We agreed I'd stay with our bikes and Bob would return to meet me. I waited and watched, looking expectantly in the direction he'd gone, but somehow he slipped by my eagle eye. After twenty anxious minutes I was pacing. I left a note on Bob's bicycle seat, locked the bike, and went off in search of him, grumbling to myself.

My hopes were dashed when he wasn't at the hotel. I started to beat myself up for being so stupid as I prepared to pedal the streets. I was trying not to cry when Heiner arrived with Bob in tow. Disoriented, Bob couldn't remember the way back to the market. He also couldn't remember where we were staying, having forgotten the hotel's card. It was only by luck that Heiner found him wandering in the night market, pushing someone else's bike, thinking it was his. We returned the bike, praying Bob remembered where he'd gotten it, although I seriously doubted it. I tried not to think of the anguish it would cause if we left it in the wrong place - Heiner's bike had been stolen two days before and he'd had to pay the company for a new one.

These partial memory lapses were hard to grasp. Bob could remember he had a bike, but not where he'd parked it or where he was to meet me. He knew he was with Heiner and me, but couldn't remember the hotel we were staying in. This made taking care of him even more challenging, for we never knew what he'd remember and what he'd forget.

I realized that if I wanted to continue to travel, I'd have to adapt. I began to make sure that Bob always carried a copy of his passport, our business card, the address of the hotel where we were staying, and important phone numbers in case something should happen to me, plus a note explaining that he had Alzheimer's.

I also always made sure Bob had some money on him - enough to feel dignified, but not so much that it would hurt if he lost it. Not only did he routinely misplace it, but he couldn't tell what it was worth. Even at home in Bali, he could no longer tell the difference between an Indonesian 1000 rupiah note (worth about ten cents) and a 100,000 rupiah note (worth about ten dollars). I was constantly trying to maintain a delicate balance, tottering between being too helpful and not being helpful enough, afraid of leaving him out on a limb to deal with a situation he couldn't handle.

We'd been in Luang Prabang for six days and were on our way to meet Heiner for afternoon coffee when I popped into an Internet place to take a quick peek at e-mail. Bob promised he'd sit on the bench outside to people-watch – still one of his favorite pastimes. But he soon came in and said he'd just walk to the end of the block a few yards away. I was in the middle of an important e-mail to our staff back in Bali, so I reluctantly said, "Alright, but just to the end of the block and then come right back." When I went outside, he was nowhere in sight.

Heading towards the designated cafe, I met Heiner.

"I've lost him again!"

I was feeling pretty stupid at this point. We both hoped Bob would be at the cafe. He wasn't. Rain was immanent. Hoping

Bob would magically appear, we ordered coffee while the rain poured down. Soon it was dark.

Back at the hotel we found him locked out of our room. He'd left his key inside and hadn't thought to ask the staff to open it for him. He was depressed. The afternoon's experience had made him realize how much his memory had decayed. "I wonder how long until you put me away?" he said sadly.

***

I was finding that being a caregiver was a constant dance with the disease, a constant letting go of what I held sacred, of what I thought was important for my own mental health, such as having 'morning alone' time. Being creative is a necessity for me, not an option, but oddly I found Alzheimer's could be an outlet for creativity as well.

Back in Bali I started finding interesting ways to keep me on track. I'd scan the BBC online for neutral or positive news I could bring to the breakfast table so we had something to talk about rather than sitting in silence. News of wars, politics, or violence upset Bob, so I'd steer clear of those topics. Not only did I learn a lot - *did you realize that dinosaurs roamed the earth for 165 million years?* - but I'd use the articles to stimulate conversation. Alzheimer's had taken away Bob's ability to initiate conversation or just chat. Most of his references were to his distant past, rarely to our twenty-four years together. Before dementia, we'd always had plenty to say to one another. I missed this part of our relationship.

For me, keeping a travel journal had always been a good way to relive a trip. Months or years later, I'd bring one to the table and read an entry or two after each meal. Those journals and I became Bob's memory – we'd take the journey once again at the dining table on the verandah overlooking our tropical garden. This, like the news stories, gave us topics to discuss, laugh about and break the Alzheimer's silence.

Traveling or not, I found that if Bob had something to consult regarding our schedule for the day, he'd be less anxious and I wouldn't have to answer the same questions repeatedly. I came up with a form with spaces for the date and the day of the week and a list of what we were doing at what time. If the list wasn't absolutely accurate, it didn't matter because he wouldn't notice the holes in the schedule or remember what I'd elaborated on, but having this small piece of paper seemed to ease his mind. He'd consult it several times a day provided it was out where he'd see it.

***

To celebrate my sixtieth birthday in 2006 I wanted to return to Italy one last time with Bob. I knew our traveling days were numbered, but I thought I'd learned enough from previous trips to handle whatever might arise. With the Laos lessons still fresh in my memory we met our dear friend Marisa in Venice. Marisa had a soft spot for Bob, who reminded her of her late father.

Driving was in Bob's blood and he was still good at it as long as we did the navigating. We rented a car and toured through Northern Tuscany. He maneuvered through narrow cobblestoned roads passing through villages where the buildings on opposite sides of the streets were only separated by a single lane. Bob did brilliantly, keeping up with the Italian drivers, but I think it also gave us false hope that he wasn't as badly off as we'd thought.

The day of my birthday Marisa took him off to a museum to give me some alone time. She told me later, "Susan, he's so dependent on you! Even though I kept telling him we'd see you soon, he was continually asking where you were. It was a shock for me to realize what this disease has done to him."

I knew he'd become totally dependent on me, but it was unnerving to have it mirrored back. On the one hand, when we were all together he almost seemed normal – joking, sipping wine, enjoying his meals, and following us around Venice on and off the *vaporetti*. He could also still take care of his physical and grooming needs. Then reality would step in and we'd see that he couldn't survive in Venice by himself for even a few hours. It was our last vacation together.

Chapter Sixteen
Coming Loose

Do not go where the path may lead
Go instead where there is no path
And leave a trail.

- Ralph Waldo Emerson

The early years of living with Alzheimer's were challenging, but I kept thinking, *I can do this!* Like a frog put into pot of cool water with the heat slowly increased, I hardly noticed it was getting hotter. But a slowly-heated frog ends up being boiled to death, and at times I thought that's what Alzheimer's was doing to me. Still, I persevered, in spite of the occasional meltdown.

Bob was having increasing problem-solving difficulties and a hard time remembering instructions in the workshop. Besides designing jewelry, we also designed sculptures out of mammoth tusk. They ranged from Buddhas and Kuan Yins to cheetah families and elephants or frogs chasing flies. Bob made the wood bases for our sculptures and sometimes also used large crystals we'd purchased on our annual trips to India. I would go over each sculpture to explain what I wanted and he'd grind the crystal and make a hole for the pin so it would sit right on the rock. For the wood, he'd form the bases using a band saw, grinder, and sander to get the shape I'd requested.

As the disease progressed, he couldn't keep track of his tools and got angry if I patiently tried to explain, for the umpteenth time, what I wanted for a particular base. "You're treating me like a child!" he'd roar, slamming down whatever was in his hand. Soon, he could no longer keep the instructions straight and would come back to me repeatedly, asking the same questions over and over, interrupting the flow of my work. I devised a paper form for each sculpture, with room for the instructions, drawings, dimensions, and the date. This solution succeeded for a year and a half. But by 2005, it became clear that Bob couldn't continue making the bases for our sculptures. My instructions stopped making sense because he couldn't remember what he'd read at the top of the form by the time he got to the bottom. I hired a new man to replace him before it was too late for Bob to pass on his workshop knowledge.

As Bob's ability to work weakened, I took over more and more of our business. I also made lists for Bob and posted notes with my whereabouts on the front door with the hour I could be expected back and my cell phone number underlined, should he need to contact me. I later found my number in his handwriting all over the house - in notebooks, in his drawer, in his wallet. He knew I was his lifeline.

***

Over the years, Bob had done most of the packing for our various trips, but gradually I had to take that job over too.

He'd fill his suitcase with unnecessary items such as socks that he never wore in the tropics, too many pairs of pants, and no underwear, or only one shirt for a three-week trip. A silent battle ensued where I'd remove the unnecessaries, replacing them with things he needed, and he'd refill the suitcase with more and different items when I wasn't looking.

This was all happening in the midst of our busy lives. While my White Knight and Protector was falling apart, I was taking over his role. I tried to think ahead, looking out for what might befall him. I kept track and possession of all the important papers like our passports, checks, and ATM cards. I made lists and notes from previous trips so I'd know what to look out for, such as noting he could no longer fill in, by himself, the immigration forms necessary to enter a country and that I needed to be patient with him. I made notes of what he needed for clothes and toiletries for each place we regularly visited. I was a list keeper, so this all came naturally and helped me feel less insecure about caring for him while traveling.

Although Bob was still driving, he couldn't navigate without me, getting completely lost if he went out on his own. The time that finally drove this home to me happened when he'd gone to get the car washed and shop for a few items at the grocery store. Anxiously watching the clock tick away the hours, I started making contingency plans about what to do if he didn't come back. Miraculously, he drove up the driveway, but with a look of terror on his face and the car strewn with maps he couldn't make sense of. Soon after that, he had a few near misses and it became evident that driving was the next piece of his identity to be yanked away, and with it another part of his dignity.

***

The Tucson Gem and Mineral Show remained one of our main sources of income. We not only sold our work there, but also bought supplies to take back to Bali. By 2006 Bob had become so anxious and irritable that he could hardly stand still, constantly organizing and reorganizing boxes in the booth. Ginia, our saleswoman, pulled me aside. "Susan, Bob can't cope with the pressure of selling or finding stock or putting it away anymore. He's often angry at me, or worse, the customers."

I was just about to enter the booth after a bathroom break the following day when I heard a customer steaming, "I will never buy from that man again!" as he stomped off. We realized I'd have to find someone to care for Bob the following year.

So in 2007 his daughters agreed to share care of him while I did the exhibitions with our friend Heiner filling in for Bob. But less than a week after we arrived in California, my husband complained of a backache, refused dinner, and by morning had developed a high fever. I thought he had the flu.

I returned from doing errands to find him half on and half off the bed, unable to move, and babbling nonsense. The ER doctor ran tests and concluded he had both encephalitis, an acute inflammation of the brain, and viral spinal meningitis. The doctor also told me the Alzheimer's would be more advanced if Bob survived. I could hardly breathe. The idea that Bob would suddenly be worse was unfathomable. I didn't even contemplate the idea that he might not survive.

Bob's daughters came to be with him, allowing me to do the Tuscon exhibitions. We needed the money more than ever, not knowing how much of the medical costs would be covered by insurance. And Heiner was a Godsend. I couldn't do the shows without a man to do the lifting and help erect the booths. He generously rolled up his sleeves and got busy, and with his well-organized German background, the setting up and taking down of the booths was more efficient than ever. He also gave me a shoulder to cry on and emotional support to get through the show.

Our friends and family sent good wishes, healing energy and prayers from all over the world. Many people waited for my frequent emails to hear how Bob was doing, showing me how much love was in our lives. Every day I called his room from Tucson. But when he awoke from a five-day coma, he was not the man who went into it.

***

There was snow on the ground when I returned to the hospital in California after three weeks away. Bob had spent twelve days in acute care and was now in the rehabilitation unit learning to eat, walk, and speak again. When I walked into his room, the nurses were trying to get him up, but he was having trouble following their instructions. He needed a haircut and beard trim, and had a wild, crazed look in his eyes.

Suddenly, he said, "I need to pee. Now!" and got up, wobbly, on his own. I steadied him until he bolted for the toilet door and peed all over the seat. It felt like a major accomplishment that he'd gotten there by himself.

In the evening, as I was preparing to go, he said, "Don't go. I'm scared here." His pleading brought tears that I tried to push back. My stomach tightened. I felt so badly leaving and yet I desperately needed the increasingly elusive state of sleep. I'd lie awake in the wee hours, my mind a whirr of thoughts and emotions.

Once he was up, walking around and able to feed himself, Bob was irascible and willfully resistant to any form of aid. Thin before the illness, he'd lost twenty-one pounds and looked like a scarecrow in his clothes. He was also incontinent.

The rehab unit wasn't accustomed to dementia patients and didn't know how to handle him. He wandered into other patients' rooms, taking things or leaving a pile of poop in a corner. He scurrilously refused help with showering and resisted going into the bathroom altogether unless it was his own idea. And he frequently tried to escape out of the door by the nurse's station, especially at night when he couldn't sleep and roamed the halls in the early hours trying to find someone to talk with him. For Bob, night and day had merged into Now. His doctor, nurses and caseworker all counseled me, "You can't take him home. You'll never be able to manage him alone." I knew they were right. I wasn't strong enough to handle his weight if he fell. And how would I avoid sleep deprivation when he was up half the night?

Bob had become combative if he sensed he was being controlled by anyone, including me. I wasn't ready to give up and stow him in a place where I'd only be able to visit two months of the year, yet I had to keep our business running. I knew I couldn't take care of him in his present condition and work at the same time. "We think it would be best to find an Alzheimer unit to place Bob in," the caseworker said, handing me a list of available homes in the area.

Reluctantly, I visited one of the residential units. The cheerfulness of the woman who greeted me in the lobby annoyed me profusely. The décor was little-old-lady-prints and soft colors; the background music could have been borrowed from a department store. I so did not want to be there. When the staff offered me tea and cookies, the sight of them made me nauseous.

The odor that greeted me when we stepped through the door to the lockdown Alzheimer's unit was a mixture of body fluids and pine-scented cleanser. Four elderly women in various stages of dementia were playing cards with a caregiver. A man was endlessly walking the length of the room and back. I dutifully looked at rooms, some single, some shared. A few had people in them, and I felt I was invading their private space, but at their stage of Alzheimer's, there was no private space. The rooms were all depressing. There were no upbeat tropical colors like those in our house in Bali, and no verdant garden to keep Bob busy. I couldn't see him surviving there for long. He'd probably never recognize me again if I left him there. He'd go stark raving mad, and if he didn't, I would, knowing I'd put him away.

I followed the tour guide back to the office and looked over the price list. The base price wasn't too bad, but every pill that needed to be administered, every adult diaper changed, any help with feeding in the future, anything and everything that Bob needed help with would add to the cost. Our savings would be gone in less than two years. *And then what?*

Back in the car, I sat behind the wheel, sobbing. There was no way I could put Bob in a place like this, but I couldn't deal with incontinence or sleep deprivation for long and I had to keep working to put food on the table. I felt lost, unable to see beyond the fog of life with Alzheimer's.

Bob's daughters and I agreed that none of us were ready to leave him in the care of an institution. "Why don't you move in with me until Dad's well enough to return to Bali?" Dawn suggested. We believed he'd get better faster in a loving atmosphere surrounded by his grandchildren. Six weeks after he went into the hospital, we drove him seven hours to Dawn's house in central California without mishap.

The doctors had told us that the symptoms caused by encephalitis would improve over the next year but we'd have no way to tell where his brain's recovery from this trauma would meet the continuing decline of Alzheimer's. Meanwhile, we were scrambling to keep him safe. We had an adult two-year-old who needed constant monitoring so that he didn't put a handful of pistachio nuts, shell and all, into his mouth, or drink paint water from his granddaughter's art projects. Newly installed door alarms warned us of his attempted escapes and we couldn't leave him alone for longer than a few minutes. Slowly, his long-term memory came back as he started to remember more of his past. A cognitive therapist, a physical therapist, and a nurse came to the house several times a week to continue his rehabilitation, giving me much-needed breaks. Fortunately, the incontinence mostly abated. We also enrolled Bob in adult daycare so I could have seven hours of uninterrupted work twice a week.

Christina, the angel who ran the daycare center, tried her hardest to integrate Bob into the camaraderie, but he hated it. He refused to enter into group activities, separating himself by sitting alone in the garden.

One morning a group of church ladies came to look at the premises to see if they wanted to raise funds for improvements as a community project. Bob was feeling tired and cranky, and had gone to lie down in the nap room. While Christina was giving the visitors a tour, she glanced into an alcove and there was Bob, stark naked. She carefully extracted herself from the church ladies and steered Bob away undetected, but he soon escaped to the kitchen and started masturbating.

My first reaction, "Oh my God, Christina, I'm horrified!" erupted into a belly laugh. It was like a scene from an adult sit-com. I felt it was Bob's way of saying, "I hate this place! I don't want to be here!"

Over the next month and a half, he steadily improved, but I was exhausted and foggy-brained from tracking him day and night and trying to work. I'd feel I was handling the stress, and then something minor would happen, like stubbing my toe, and I'd crumple on the floor into a pile of tears. Dawn took it all in her stride and acted as a stabilizing force.

I was desperate for intelligent conversation about spirit, creativity, and travel, and greatly missed having a partner to solve problems, plan, and reminisce with. *I want my soulmate!* I shouted to the moon. He'd disappeared, leaving me with a familiar stranger inhabiting his body. I knew it was impossible to bring him back, but still I longed for it. I tried to assuage these feelings by telling myself, *At least I have a partner to share the moment with, even though our perceptions of the moment are radically different.*

***

Our twenty-first anniversary in 2007 brought back a kaleidoscope of memories: the white horse-drawn carriage, the lacy sea-foam dress secretly hidden away until the ceremony, our family and friends blessing the rings, and Bob so handsome in his peach silk shirt and tie, beaming me up the aisle with eyes of happiness.

Our anniversary day was warm and sunny, with a clear blue sky - a perfect day for lunch at Pete's Pierside Café with gulls and pelicans and fat blubbery sea lions belching out their calls. As we waited for our food, six pelicans flew over us, quickening my heart, reminding me of the epiphany at age sixteen that had changed my life forever. That experience had been real-beyond-real, and so intense that I'd spent decades trying to understand it, and trying to experience the sensation again.

Having a Pelican Day opened me up to the joy Bob and I still shared when we were relaxed together and I wasn't trying to do five things at once. I felt that the essential Bob, the Bob at his core, and that part of me were deeply connected. I couldn't turn away from that. If a crystal ball had shown me the Alzheimer's future on our wedding day, I wouldn't have changed anything. Bob was still my Sweet Wonderful Man and I still loved him voraciously. Even though I received a lot of feedback from well-meaning friends telling me that Bob was gone, I knew he was still in there. At his core he was still the same person. I couldn't abandon him.

I hoped, in the coming year, I'd make peace with the world he was inhabiting and learn to enjoy his perpetual present moment without needing him to see things from my perspective. It was a tall wish.

***

After six weeks with Dawn, Bob was strong enough for the flight back to Bali. He'd regained his balance and part of his strength, but he could no longer lift our heavy bags of mammoth tusk, equipment, and beads. Dawn's boyfriend agreed to accompany us on the long flight home to help with the luggage and watch Bob when I needed to use the restroom. He was another angel who touched our lives, making the exhausting trip manageable.

Our staff welcomed us with a flower-filled house, but were shocked by Bob's deterioration. Nothing felt the same. Yet I was delighted to be home again.

In the years we'd lived in Bali, Bob had always done the driving. The narrow, potholed roads were dangerous. Animals and children darted out unexpectedly and motorbike drivers turned into traffic without looking to see what was bearing down on them. After encephalitis, Bob could no longer drive, and I couldn't envision a future being dependent on anyone else. We were home only a few days when I took to the wheel.

In Indonesia, vehicles are driven on the left side of the road, so making the switch to changing gears with the other hand was a challenge. As I reached the main street in our aging van, I struggled to turn without power steering and hit a rock that was protecting a tree. Embarrassed, I backed up, straightened out and kept going with a wildly pounding heart. It took me a week to find the courage to get out of second gear.

Bob didn't understand why he wasn't driving. "Honey, you've been driving me all over Bali for seventeen years. Now it's my turn to drive you!" We got a laugh out of that line, day after day, month after month.

The move home confused my sweet husband, especially at night. He'd get up several times and flash a light around, trying to figure out where he was, waking me in the course of these discovery trips or when he was trying to find the bathroom. He had a hard time not getting tangled in the mosquito net, and I caught him several times trying to pee on the wall. Like the mother of a small child, I became increasingly aware of his every move in the night, my ears always cocked for trouble. Lack of sleep crept up on me. I tried giving Bob Valium, but then he got up drugged and was even more difficult to deal with.

Some of our friends assumed I was miserable. "You must feel imprisoned," said one. I could see that, from the outside, our life looked frightening. But from inside it simply felt like life doing its thing. There was nothing to do but live to the best of our ability. I was learning to let go of my fantasy of how I wanted my life to be, to let go of my mate being there for me, and to let go of security.

And hardest of all, I was learning to let go of my ego... me, me, me. I realized that Bob's comfort had to come first. I'm not saying I denied my feelings – all the emotions were right there, but thanks to Ramesh's teachings, I saw them as just emotions arising in response to a thought. They were no longer so damned personal. I still cried, laughed, got angry, experienced the whole gamut of feelings, but it was as if they were happening in the next room rather than occupying the center of my vision. Making our world focus around Bob actually made my life easier because he was happier. Since he had lost the ability to consider others, I couldn't expect give and take.

Pre-Alzheimer's, Bob had been very supportive of me; now it was my turn to take care of him. At times I still fell into the trap of old behaviors, like expecting he would clean up if I cooked or being irritable if he interrupted my concentration, but I accepted that they too were part of this journey. On the upside, I had work I loved, supportive friends, and moments when the curtain parted and there was a connection with Bob. That connection was especially strong when we danced.

We liked to go to Jazz Café, one of the few cafes in Ubud with live music. Never shy about being first, we enjoyed having the dance floor to ourselves. We'd look deeply into each other's eyes as the spark between us ignited with the steps and the beat of the music. Bob was now so uninhibited that I had to parry his hungry hands with deft moves to keep us from 'dirty dancing'.

One evening we returned to our table to be greeted by a waiter bearing a bottle of champagne. "We didn't order this," I said, embarrassed.

"It's a gift from that table over there." He pointed to a couple we'd never seen before. The salt-and-pepper haired man was dressed casually but elegantly. The woman was all bundled up with a wide-brimmed polka dot hat and an orange sarong around her shoulders. She had a stiff look of pain about her and a bandage on her chin, and was sitting exceedingly still in this room filled with Latin rhythms.

We danced over to them. "Thank you so much for the bubbly. It was very kind of you. But we're curious why you sent it."

The man took my hand, kissed it, and said in a sensual French accent, "The way you look into your husband's eyes when you dance touches my heart." Later, we saw his companion walk with painful difficulty to the ladies room. When she returned, her partner danced solo for her in an elfin way, full of life, keeping eye contact with her as he tried to take her mind off her condition to show his love.

***

The challenge of caring for Bob had escalated in the wake of encephalitis. Citalopram, an anti-depressant, helped smooth his anxiety and irritability, making life easier for both of us. Anti-depressants, often prescribed by doctors for Alzheimer's patients, help control their high level of anxiety, but it can take months, as it did for us, to get the right dosage. Give too much and you have a zombie on your hands, sleepy and in danger of falling, and without enough, the anxiety is still there, coloring the air with agitation.

As the effects of the brain inflammation wore off, Bob became completely self-absorbed. He still had manners. He'd ask, "How are you?" but there wasn't any follow-up if the person didn't say, "Fine". When I told him that Helen had lost her fifteen-year battle with cancer, his reaction was a flat, "We all have to die." He didn't ask for details, or how Lisa was coping. His world had been whittled down to a kernel of survival.

Sometimes a vague insecurity enveloped him. "Where do we live?" "Whose names are the cars registered under?" "What if one of us dies?" I knew what he really meant was "What if Susan dies?" In spite of the vast range of things Bob couldn't remember, somewhere inside he knew I was his lifeline.

Bob's queries brought up questions of my own. I didn't know how to plan for our future, having no idea how the disease would continue to unfold for him. Bob sometimes didn't even know who I was, or that something was wrong with him. He'd even forgotten that his mother and two of her sisters had died of the same disease. Bob was sequestered deeply inside himself, looking at the world through the bars of Alzheimer's with the shade pulled down.

The following year, on our last trip together to the States, my denial about Bob's ability to travel dissolved. We were staying with my sister, Joan. "I'm going out front to sweep the driveway," Bob said. It was five o'clock on a warm March afternoon.

"Ok. But come right back in when you're done." What was I thinking? He'd never remember that instruction.

About an hour later, Joan and I were inside, chatting and sipping a cocktail. Lost in conversation, we'd forgotten the time. "Oh my God, Joan! Where's Bob?" I croaked when I looked at the clock. We dashed outside, but there was only his broom, propped up against a shrub. We went off on foot to search for him.

Our first stop was Joan's next door neighbors. "Oh, I thought he must live around here somewhere,' said the husband. "He wandered into our house, into the bedroom where I was lying down. At first I was shocked, especially when he insisted this was his house and wanted to know what I was doing here. But I soon realized he was no threat, just confused. So I walked him to the door and tried to point him towards your house. I wasn't even sure that's where he needed to go. I didn't realize he had dementia."

After a thorough search of the neighborhood by car, Joan and I came up empty-handed and called the police. They brought Bob back to us a few hours later. He'd realized he was lost and had walked into a veterinary clinic over a mile away, telling them he needed help.

***

Since we'd been living in Bali, Bob and I had welcomed our regular visa runs. They brought pauses from work when we could explore new territory, revisit favorite places, or connect with the many friends we'd made over the years. After the mishap at my sister's, I realized that Bob would have to get a retirement visa so he could stay in Bali without having to leave the island on a regular basis. He wouldn't be returning to the States. But there would have to be one more trip outside of Indonesia to get that needed visa – a trip that would see my worst fear manifested. Bangkok, where we had friends, a doctor and dentist, and a small amount of business to do, seemed a good choice.

We were used to walking long distances when we traveled, but at seventy-five, Bob could no longer keep up. He often stumbled, and if a bathroom wasn't near, he'd wet his pants. This gallant man was then reduced to walking down the street with a large wet spot front and center. When I finally managed to get him into incontinence underwear, I was relieved but battle weary. The constant monitoring and the fear that I wouldn't be able to keep him safe undid me.

Then the fear of all fears transpired. We'd just made our way through the thick crowd descending from the Sky Train in a hyper-busy part of Bangkok. People were pushing past us in their world of hurry. Bob always walked a few paces behind me to keep me in his vision, never alongside me anymore or in front. We were weaving in and out of the crowd when I turned, as I always did, to check that he was still following. Searing panic shot through my body. There was no Bob in sight! I was about to cry when some inner strength grabbed hold of me and sternly declared: *No! Crying is not helpful right now!*

I rushed back to the bottom of the Sky Train stairs, but he wasn't there. I felt nauseous. Bangkok is a huge metropolis. How would I ever find him? I knew he wouldn't remember the name of our hotel and wouldn't have a clue how to find me.

Then a miracle happened. Bob wandered back to the stairs with a look of terror on his face. I was so relieved I wasn't even angry. I knew in that instant that we'd never travel anywhere together again. Good-bye to another piece.

Chapter Seventeen
Obsessions and Distractions

This once together
Disciplined woman
Has fired the guard of her inner sanctum
Flung the doors open
To be ravished by magnetic words
Whispered across the Atlantic

Not long after we returned from Bangkok, I left Bob with Nyoman, who'd been driving for us on the long errand trips down south after encephalitis took Bob's driving ability away. Nyoman was a quiet man, grounded and substantial, though he had a boyish face and dry sense of humor. Over time, he also became our part-time gardener and surreptitious Bob minder. I'd send him and Bob off to do invented errands in the afternoons when I needed a break. At other times I'd go for a massage or to meet a friend while they stayed home and gardened. As long as Nyoman was working or doing something useful, Bob accepted him and didn't feel he was being minded. But after a while, the situation grew taut.

Re-energized from a coffee date, I entered the gate to the garden. Nyoman was nowhere to be seen - not a good sign. Bob was rummaging around in the house alone. Finally, Nyoman appeared. "Bob very angry at Nyoman," he said shyly. "Sent me away and yelled, 'I don't need you to look after me! Go home!' I know Bob doesn't mean it. But it hurt. I stayed near the car so I could watch, make sure he was safe".

I plunked down on the sofa, dreading what I was hearing. My throat constricted as gentle Nyoman lowered his gaze. "I've thought of quitting. But I don't want to leave you alone."

When he told me how often Bob was angry, tears spilled over. I didn't know how I'd bear it if Nyoman quit. He gave me the only respite I got, an hour or two here or there to have some time without Alzheimer's in my face.

Our other staff confirmed how often Bob was irritable. He frequently accused them of stealing his broom, shoes, or scoop. I was facing the possibility that soon I might not be able to handle my husband. I'd imagined I'd be able to find people to take care of him as his disease progressed. Now, I wasn't so sure. But I couldn't abide what that might mean, so I pushed the thought away.

A month later, Nyoman reluctantly told me, "I think I can earn more money as a freelance driver. My brother-in-law, Rudy, would like the job. His father is confused too, so he understands." I was crestfallen.

Rudy, a far cry from Nyoman, stopped by the next day. He was now the only hope of respite I had. He wasn't as sharp as Nyoman, I had to take longer with instructions, and he lacked the initiative his brother-in-law had. He took over gardening with Bob and I'd send the two of them off to run errands after I explained to Bob how much I valued his opinion in choosing the right products so he'd go without a fuss. It was getting more and more difficult to convince him to go. Rudy made himself busy so it didn't look like he was a minder, but he really wasn't suited for the job.

It seemed whenever I got respite, it was quickly ripped away. One day I came home after a few glorious, creative hours in my studio to find Bob again locked in the house and Rudy hiding out by the car. Bob had become angry and sent him to pull nails out of non-existent wood supposedly stored by our vehicle, then gone inside and locked the door. When I entered the house, I found Bob reorganizing his jewelry, which he often did, only this time he'd gotten into mine as well. He'd bagged necklaces and rings and bracelets and written notes wanting to know who made them and when, and the costs. All the jewelry was mixed up. It would take days to relocate missing pieces. I lost control and yelled at him, then fled in tears to the bathroom, where I was getting well-acquainted with the floor tiles.

Other times I'd return from a respite break and be faced with a flooded kitchen that Rudy had missed because he was trying to stay in the background, or the stove lit with no pot or pan on the burner. Bob was adamant that he didn't need a minder and was perfectly capable of caring for himself. In trying to stay out of the line of fire, Rudy missed some of Bob's misadventures. He, too, was growing weary of anger directed at him. Rudy barely lasted a year.

***

In 2009, my fortitude cracked, revealing my outermost limits. My can't-take-any-more wall loomed up on the horizon.

I realized I'd been barely hanging on for so long that it felt like the new normal. I was desperate for respite from the Alz grind and the accumulated stress that comes with the disease.

Bob continued to be angry much of the time. He was sure that someone was stealing from him or watching him. I finally realized he needed more care than we could provide. It was too disruptive for the staff running our business to try to watch over him too. I placed an ad in the local paper and told anyone who'd listen that I was looking for caregivers to train.

The grapevine brought us Ketut, who'd cared for an Australian writer confined to a wheelchair, a man who'd been completely dependent on his caregivers but still had a brilliant mind. Ketut was comfortable caring for someone whose body had given out, but dealing with the challenges of Bob's deteriorating mind brought him new tests of patience. Nano came with no experience in caregiving, but was eager to learn, and his English was better than Ketut's. At first they trained together in the afternoons and early evenings as they learned how to deal with Bob. As time and the disease progressed and their confidence increased, they worked longer shifts, each on their own. They invented clever 'tricks' or ways to deal with Bob that would cause him the least anxiety.

"Hey Bob, I need your help with my English. I have letter to write," Ketut said one day, just as Bob was about to wield a machete on a stand of bamboo. The last time he'd gotten hold of that sickle, it had resulted in eight stitches in his left hand. Someone had left it out of its hiding place. Thankfully, this time Bob dropped the machete and went to help Ketut, completely forgetting the knife. Later, Ketut put it out of sight. Out of sight was usually out of mind for Bob.

I pinned all my respite hopes on these bright, patient men, even though Bob was not so eager to accept them into his life. But soon after, I came home one afternoon from an art opening, happy to have had some respite and artistic inspiration, only to find Bob locked inside the house again with the windows closed and the shades lowered. Nano and Ketut were sitting outside.

"Bob was helping me with my English," Nano explained. "But then it started raining. He got anxious and went into the house and locked us out."

It was five in the afternoon, sundowner's time, a difficult time for many Alz people, who are affected by the dimming light. I couldn't unlock the door because Bob had his key in the lock on the inside. I was red-faced livid. Of course, Bob didn't remember doing this and said snottily, "Well, they could have knocked," when I asked why he'd locked out his carers.

My equilibrium was giving out and I was sleep deprived.

"What're you doing? It's one in the morning!" I wailed.

Bob was beaming a strong flashlight around the room. "I think I spilled popcorn on the floor."

"Get back in bed, Bob. We've never eaten popcorn in this house." I was too tired to remember not to correct him. He got up five times more, waking me with each episode. I woke in a morning fog to the sound of grunting. Bob was peeling pillowcases off the pillows, looking for money. He looked at me imploringly. "Do I have any clothes here? Are we leaving this place today?"

During this period, the anti-depressants that kept his anxiety at a manageable level ran out. The doctor in America wouldn't prescribe more unless he saw Bob, but the thirty-hour trip would have done us in. The only way I could ever take him back to the States would be to have help, and then to leave him there. I was still not prepared to consider that possibility.

We couldn't get the same drug in Indonesia so we started the process of finding a substitute. We went through two months of torment trying to find a replacement and dosage that was successful.

Out one evening at an Italian film festival, I got a panicked call from Ketut. "Bob's gone walkabout." He'd become agitated and wanted to play with the dogs in the street. Ketut was keeping an eye on him, but then Bob started walking and became angry about being followed.

"Bob, let's go home," Ketut had appealed. "Susan's waiting for you." But Bob put his fingers in his ears and stomped away. When I caught up with him, he was at the darkened, closed market in the center of town, and he was disoriented. Ketut was standing guard off to the side so Bob wouldn't see him.

Ketut told me, "Yesterday afternoon, Bob thought two men were after him. He threw his broom and scoop over the garden wall. Then he hid in the back corner of the garden. He wouldn't listen to me." We changed drugs.

The next anti-depressant we tried made him zombiesque and incontinent. Another had him so relaxed he tripped and fell, doing a header into the fishpond. My staff and I were frantically trying to run the business and keep watch over Bob until Nano and Ketut started their late afternoon shift. Being responsible for Bob was exhausting all of us. It was during this time that the Alz angels, Hanna and Keith, came to our rescue after reading an ad I'd put in the local paper looking for caregivers. Keith was a retired doctor who'd specialized in geriatric medicine while his partner, Hanna, was a retired caseworker specializing in supporting caregivers of dementia patients. They were living in the next village for six months. With their expertise in caring for people with dementia, they trained the three of us how to live with Bob in the best way possible. We learned not to correct him, to let him be right. We learned to hone our skills at redirection so Bob was steered away from a potentially dangerous direction into a positive one while thinking it was his decision. We also learned to distinguish when Bob was speaking and when the disease was.

The Angels came at the right time. I wept when their font of knowledge cascaded over me, soothing my worries, fears, and sadness. They were so wise and compassionate that I felt scooped up and enfolded in their benevolent wings, even when I was seven thousand miles away in Italy.

Keith helped with drug choices if needed, and ways to circumvent behavioral problems without them. He explained how to tell the difference between delusional behavior and dementia, the first a common sign there's something wrong, such as an infection that the patient isn't even aware of or can't articulate. "Delusion is seeing chickens in the room. Dementia is not being sure how many there are."

Hanna taught us to become masters of redirection, to understand the disease and use Bob's voracious sweet tooth. When he went off on one of his compulsive tangents, such as being obsessed with the car that he could no longer drive, we learned to call to him, "There's a cookie waiting for you in the kitchen, Bob." We'd see him immediately change direction. By the time he reached the kitchen, he'd forgotten both the car and the cookie.

***

Periodically, my sweet husband became soft and romantic, "What a great life we have," he told me one day. I reached for his hand and he looked into my eyes. "You're beautiful, and I'm so happy being with you." My heart began to melt. Places he used to inhabit inside of me softened, yearning. Then my armor clanked closed. I couldn't feel anything but numb. *I hate this!"* I yelled inside, pushing against the paralysis I felt. *Why can't I just be open to him the way he is?*

I had such compassion for Bob, but letting him touch me romantically was just too excruciating. I didn't have the courage to endure the pain left behind when my hope that our connection was still alive was dashed once again. But every once in a while I'd forget this and allow his advances to continue. Since the encephalitis, Bob had lived in a constant disconnect, but I didn't, and occasionally a temporary 'caregiver amnesia' would take over. Or was it wishful thinking?

My shutting down didn't go away. Was it the constancy of the disease? Anger? The repetitions? The lack of sleep? I questioned myself mercilessly, trying to find something solid to base my feelings on. Friends who were willing to hear me rant or vent or cry became my lifeline and kept me sane. "How much longer can you do this, Susan?" they asked.

Margie, who was by now my closest friend, gave me sage insights that helped me understand what I was really feeling and helped me not to feel guilty for whatever came up. She was also the Queen of Silly, and sometimes we squealed and giggled in our own world until Bob shouted, "Will you two shut up!" as though we were annoying children.

My sister, Joan, and I emailed each other every day, and no matter how much I whined, she was always willing to listen and give me a fresh perspective. Her love was like tree roots, keeping my ground stable. Heiner, who'd rescued me in 2007 by coming to help me at Tuscon while Bob was hospitalized with encephalitis, stopped by for hugs and to joke with Bob. He brought sweets. I made him espresso. Our neighbors and close friends, Jean and William, listened to my ruminations. They, and my friend, Victoria, tried to help me keep the situation in perspective, questioning my resolve to push on for fear I'd hurt myself. And Cat, a wise, objective Canadian who'd moved to Bali and become a friend a few years back, gently pushed me to see the situation from a distance and insisted that I take care of myself. She also invited me out regularly for frozen lychee martinis with a varying round of other expat women.

Having Nano and Ketut gave me a spot of respite, but instead of feeling relieved, I often saw just how stressed I was. My creativity felt clogged. Tears were always just under the surface, holding hands with anger. Bob's irritability depressed me, but what really sank me under was my ever-increasing bouts of exasperation.

These situations built until one evening, after listening to Bob abuse his caregivers once again, I couldn't hold back. "We have to talk, Bob. This is not a threat. But if you don't allow me to take care of you in the best way I know how - and that includes help from others - then I'll have no choice but to put you somewhere in America."

Bob looked lost and forlorn, but I couldn't stop.

I gathered myself in a very calm, measured manner and continued. "You just can't treat our employees this way. Nyoman quit because of the way you treated him. I have to take care of our business. I need breaks. So you'll have to get used to caregivers helping you because you can't be alone. You have Alzheimer's and you won't remember this conversation for long."

I was at breaking point. And still I knew this talk would do no good.

"Well, I guess I should just do myself in then. I'm no use to you," he said, his voice flat and his eyes downcast.

"That's not an option. And besides, you're basically pretty happy with your life. Or so you reiterate quite frequently. You just have to allow us to care for you."

Five minutes later, Bob had forgotten this exchange and was focused on a wildlife TV program. I wondered, *"How will I pull this off if he won't accept help? How can I go to Tucson to do our shows and leave him here with Nano and Ketut?*

I texted Margie: "I'm having a meltdown." She and Heiner came straight over to console me with hugs and support. Bob joined us on the veranda and said, "I don't know how I'll get home."

"This is your home, Bob," I said. "You've lived here a long time." Margie stroked his arm. Heiner, looking stunned, didn't know what to say. He was just quietly there in support, concern knitted on his brow.

Bob went in the house to get ready for bed, but five minutes later he appeared again, looking perplexed. "Which bed do I sleep in?" (We only had one.) "I haven't explored the house to get familiar with it yet."

Had my anger made him more confused? Clearly, my talk with him had done nothing for either of us. How could I avoid going down this path yet again?

Always on high alert, my senses were automatically attuned to where Bob was, what he was doing, and what he might be feeling. I was always trying to waylay problems before they arose, but new scenarios kept sneaking up and bushwhacking me. And I couldn't seem to let go of logical thinking, even though I knew full well that my sweet husband had lost the ability to be logical. Logic was so much a part of my normal functioning that, even when it was clear it wasn't working, I fell back on it anyway, especially when I was laid raw from stress.

I felt if I didn't get away soon, I'd explode.

I spent hours planning my first night away from home. Linda, my yoga teacher and long-time friend, lived in a nearby village and invited me for a trial overnight. Her house was close enough that I could get home quickly in case the caregivers needed rescuing. It would be a test to see if Nano and Ketut could handle Bob for a night. If they succeeded, we could try consecutive nights away, and then maybe I could go away for a few weeks. And then, maybe, I could go to the States to do our shows for two months. It was almost too much to hope for.

Linda gave me the best room in the house with a view of Mt. Agung in all its 10,000 feet of cloud-free splendor. Margie joined us for drinks on the veranda and then sushi and an almond flan I'd baked, knowing it was one of her favorite desserts. We laughed and giggled and got silly. It was a sanity-saving relief.

The caregivers only called once that evening, wanting to know how to turn off the computer. Bob did fine, but put a kitchen knife by the bed since I wasn't sleeping with him. Nano and Ketut were nervous about this in case he awakened scared in the night and went after them, but I knew he wouldn't remember he'd put it there.

***

As life with Bob became more and more challenging, loneliness crept in on silent cat feet, scratching at the edges of my consciousness. I didn't want to name it. I felt I'd be giving in if I spoke the word aloud. I told myself I was too busy to be lonesome. I had supportive, caring friends and a busy social life. How could I possibly be lonely? I felt weak and pathetic if I even considered it. But deep down I was awash with missing the profound connection Bob and I had shared. I missed the give and take of love, the sharing of problems and working together to solve them, the joy of intimate communion, shared memories and mealtime conversations. I missed being in love so deeply that I started fantasizing about having a lover.

My rational mind protested these daydreams, telling me a new love would complicate my already complicated life, and reminding me how guilty I'd feel. I knew what I really wanted was my soulmate back. Again, I started reading aloud at mealtimes from our old travel journals, hoping it would give Bob and I something else to talk about. The words conjured up few memories for Bob, but they gave me vivid flashbacks to how much in love we'd been.

When I'd hear Bob muttering to himself, swearing when he couldn't find an object or accomplish a task, when he'd blame anyone but himself for anything he misplaced or mismanaged, it was difficult to remember the person he'd been. The journals were a good reminder.

He was still so handsome that I loved to look at him, but since the encephalitis, the part of him that met me, joined me, and wanted to give as well as receive was gone. I kissed him, but there was no sense of him kissing me in return. My heart cried out to him, but he could no longer hear its pleas.

Alzheimer's is a self-centering disease. It leaves the person within the small box of himself. Giving is replaced by anxiety and fear. Bob was all feelings and emotions now, without understanding the consequences for him or those around him. I felt it must be horrible to be inside that box with no escape.

Like two worlds rotating on different axes, we were spinning away from one another. Bob, too, felt lonely. At three one morning he told me, "I feel so disconnected from you. You're always busy and you have your friends. We'd both be better off without me."

These references to suicide always shook me, although I knew he wouldn't remember them in the morning, so there was little danger of follow-up. I tried to be more affectionate and give him more attention. I knew I'd never stop loving him, but he'd morphed from a large male presence into a needy man-child. I longed for a man, a partner with whom I could communicate.

I continued to ask myself *Why aren't my friends enough?* But it was intimacy that I craved and diving deeper and deeper into communion. "I want my husband back!" I begged the stars, but this was a disease of silent loss that snuck up and stole the night.

***

Going through old books one day, I came upon a postcard I'd received twelve years earlier. Simone, a beau I'd had while studying Italian in Florence in 1983, had written to me at my mother's address every few years just to check in, but she'd moved, then passed away, and we'd lost contact.

When I found the card, I was curious about him and wondered how he was. I pictured him with a wife and two children. I was so sure of this picture that I believed it. He'd written on that card, 'I don't work at the post office any longer. I now sell antiques. If you and your husband are ever in Florence, I'll be your guide'. There was no return address.

Curiosity and fond memories pushed me to Google him, but I found nothing. Then, one day, I came across pages torn from an old address book I'd tossed out. His address from twenty-six years ago was there. I wrote a short note, sent a photo of one of my paintings, and enclosed a business card on the off-chance he'd not moved. I asked if he remembered me. Then, in the frenzy of Alz and 'World on a String', I forgot the whole thing until nearly a month later when sigiglio54@senza.com appeared in my inbox. I almost deleted it, thinking it was another piece of spam.

Simone wrote, 'Of course I remember you! You're my favorite artist! I've thought about you many times through the years.'

I quickly answered back.

In *Jan's Story*, Barry Peterson, who cared for his wife with early onset Alzheimer's, wrote how the darkness of the disease left him needing something to look forward to - something to take his mind off the disease. His distraction was buying and restoring old cars. Simone became mine.

Never married, Simone bought and sold antique books. He told me he liked being a bachelor and reveled in intellectual discussions about movies, music, and Tuscan cooking. His fragile, elderly mother suffered from Alzheimer's and his life revolved around her care; he saw her nearly every day, often cooking special meals for her and her live-in caregiver. This gave us an immediate connection and we commiserated about the trials and tribulations of losing a loved one to this heart-wrenching disease.

Simone's daily emails inspired me, motivating me to not lose heart. Gradually, we opened more and more to each other through the written word. Soon, innocent flirtations began, followed by lusty overtones that tendriled their way into our emails and phone calls. After months of this I was falling in love with a phantom on my monitor, bolstered by my projections of all that was missing between Bob and I. Simone was filling the gaps in my heart hacked open by Alzheimer's. He gave me a reason to wake up in the morning. He said, "You are my best friend."

I told only my closest confidants about this secret affliction. I felt I was cheating on Bob, and yet I so needed this excitement in my life, the connection, the appreciation, and the energy to fill my dangerously empty heart. I fantasized about Simone obsessively and the volume of these daydreams was so intense that at times I could hardly hear what people were saying to me. Their lips moved, but I couldn't understand the sounds. I only wanted to think about one day meeting him again.

This excitement was juxtaposed on top of the stresses of managing Bob, feeling homeless in our home, and running our business. Living largely on adrenalin, my appetite shriveled. The less sense Bob made during dining table conversations, the less food I was able to swallow. I felt full before I even sat down.

At first I was happy and proud to shed the weight since I'd spent my whole life trying to lose five to ten pounds, no matter what my weight actually was, but the pounds kept falling off. My friends became concerned. My body looked great, but my face was gaunt and the wrinkles pronounced. I looked old.

I started to use alcohol to help ease the aching reality of our shattered dream. I didn't drink every day and I tried not to drink alone, but sometimes the intensity was past bearable and I craved softer edges. Usually one gin and tonic did the trick, easing me into a 'who cares' state of mind. That was just what I wanted.

My friends told me I was funnier, happier, and more relaxed with a drink in my hand. And so The Martini Goddesses were born, a group of expat women determined to Grow Old Damned Disgracefully Every Single Second. Our meetings were often a mix of serious discussion and uproarious laughter, but at the same time we were there to support each other in difficult times and to applaud successes. This was medicine for an aching heart.

I was drinking with purpose and aware of the danger that could pose since my father had been an alcoholic. But when you reach your personal threshold of anguish, you'll do whatever is required to quell its advance, and that boundary had reached my front door.

Meanwhile, the same disease that was ripping Bob and I apart was stitching Simone and I together. We corresponded in Italian, but spoke English on the phone. I'd been studying the language again for a couple of years. Now I increased my study time, poring over lessons while I worked out at the gym.

Simone inquired frequently about Bob, gaining even more points on his scorecard with me. We shared care-giving ideas and what we'd learned about the disease, such as learning to lie without guilt to keep the person as anxiety free as possible. So if Simone's mother asked about his father, he didn't remind her he'd passed away but said he was on a business trip. As we felt each other's experience in a way none of our non-Alz-touched friends could, our openness deepened.

Simone became my muse. Paintings and poetry flowed, and

with them the idea for an artist's handmade book of poetry. I spent hours in my painting studio, creating pages in watercolor, pastel, and pencil, then scanning them into the computer along with the poetic musings that flowed from my pen. The artwork was then printed with English on the left hand page and Italian on the right.

Simone loved to cook and dreamed about having a café one day. I asked him what he'd call it. "The Wild Carrot," he said. I fantasized about having a poetry book launch at his imaginary Florentine eatery.

I was running as fast as I could away from the pain and reality of Alzheimer's, and running wildly towards a man I didn't really know. One impassioned phone call with Simone left me so raw and exposed that tears accompanied a lingering vulnerability for the rest of the day. It bordered on painful. It bordered on crazy.

As Bob grew worse, my obsession amped up. I became agitated if email was down or I couldn't reach Simone by phone. I was crazed and I knew it. I was out of control and I didn't care. *I just want the friggin' pain to stop. Now!* I told myself.

Simone fed my needs with sweet words and Italian male charm. He told me I was lovely and sexy, no matter what photo I sent, including one in my bathrobe, hair uncombed, standing in my slippers in the snow one California morning. We fantasized about traveling together, discussing movies, cooking Tuscan dishes and making love. I felt wanted and needed.

Seven months after we first connected, Simone's mother's brain could no longer command her throat to swallow, a common symptom of end stage Alzheimer's. She died a week later. Simone was overwhelmed with the necessary procedures of death, emptying her apartment, and taking care of endless Italian bureaucracy as well as grieving her loss. Distraught, he became distant. He had little time for me and said, "I probably won't be myself for at least four months."

I tried to be as understanding as possible, but once again the loneliness crept in around the craziness of every day Alz. It was accompanied by a slowly rooting idea. September was four months away. That would be a perfect time for a trip to Italy for much needed respite.

As Simone and I continued to write and talk, he realized how much I wanted to be his friend and confidante. I couldn't understand why his friends weren't more helpful and supportive when I had friends who were there for me. That should have been a red flag, but I brushed aside this sign of his distrust of people and his fierce independence. I tiptoed around him, not wanting to risk loss or confrontation. He gave me enough of a 'come on' that I moved forward with plans to visit Italy.

Just two weeks before my departure, Simone said in a phone conversation "I don't think I am who you think I am." I was floored. "We could meet for a coffee," he continued, leaving me shaking but determined to keep that out of my voice. I was grasping at a life preserver that was quickly deflating.

I made excuses for why he was treating me with indifference after leading me on with impassioned phone calls. I was drowning in fear of losing what I mistook for a thread of sanity. Or was it sanity? I started to question whether my pulling away from Bob was because of the disease, or whether my connection with this phantom that had my hibernating sexuality on high alert was luring me away. Or was it both?

After a few more trial nights away from Bob, I felt Nano and Ketut could handle whatever came up, allowing me time for a respite trip. Keith and Hanna volunteered to be on call and to take Bob out to lunch from time to time while I was away. I worked diligently to have everything in place for Bob's care, but I left for Italy an emotional mess.

In Vicenza I stayed with friends and attended a well-known jewelry trade show, trying to drum up new business and also deliver a large order to a Polish customer exhibiting there. He was so pleased with what we'd produced that he gave me more raw materials for the next order. Then, on my first day in Florence, I met a new client who bought my carvings to embellish her handmade leather bags. Things were looking up.

As I stepped through the tall wooden doors of the Renaissance building where I was staying and into a warm twilight, my phone rang. I stopped to dig it out of my handbag, barely aware of my surroundings. Simone, standing right next to me, laughed impishly as he hung up his phone. "You're more beautiful then you were twenty six years ago," he said with charming Italian aplomb.

I was trembling. I barely remembered his face after all these years and I'd forgotten we were the same height. With big blue eyes and a cleft chin, he was still cute in an awkward, boyish sort of way that belied his fifty-five years. By then I'd accepted that all we'd probably do was have a drink together with a few laughs about our Internet romance.

We fell into conversation as he led me to a bar atop a library with a so-close-it seemed-magnified view of the dome of Florence's famed Duomo. I ordered a glass of Prosecco, hoping it would take the nervousness out of my hands and voice. He ordered the same.

"Patty Smith, you know her, right? The Godmother of Punk? She just performed here – in this building," he told me as we waited for our drinks. "I saw her in a small street near here and introduced myself." Simone was always introducing himself to women in the street. That's how I'd met him in 1983 – he strode alongside me and started talking, telling me he'd seen me before and noticed the way I walked with purpose.

Our drinks came, and after a toast Simone continued. "Patty was so easy to talk to! We spoke about music and books for at least half an hour."

The story helped ease my tension; those intense blue eyes and the way his hands danced, emphasizing the story, had me entranced. "Then there was the time that Diana Krall was in town..."

"Oh, I love her music!" I interrupted.

"She's more beautiful than in her photos. And that voice! I managed to get introduced to her through a friend. Her husband, Elvis Costello, was there too." Simone winked at me and reached for my hand. I let him take it, even though I was still uncomfortable and confused by the phone call in Bali when he'd treated me with indifference.

Simone had an abundance of stories and facts about music and musicians, movies and actors, and rattled them off, filling in any silences. I realized he wasn't trying to impress me. He saw life through the filter of other people's creativity. He told me, "I feel life through music and movies more directly than I feel my own life." I wondered if this was why he had no close friends. We had a pleasant time that evening, but I realized I wasn't in love with this man, even though I was physically attracted to him. I saw clearly that the phantom on my monitor, the devil in my inbox, the sexy voice sailing through the telephone was a projection of who I'd hoped he would be, not who he really was. He'd been right, after all.

He walked me back to my room, being a bit too affectionate in public for my taste. I had to push him away a few times, but the attraction was going both ways. At my door he suggested, "Why don't you come over tomorrow and I'll cook you a traditional Tuscan lunch?

My sensible mind thought *This is dangerous territory*. My free spirit overruled and rationalized, *The man cooks. I write a recipe column for the local newspaper in Bali. Maybe I'll learn something Tuscan.*

***

I thought I disembarked from the emotional rollercoaster when I set foot on Italian soil. I thought I'd have a chance for my psyche to heal and rest before returning to the Alz fray. I thought I had better sense than to be seduced by a man living in a very messy and disorganized apartment who had only one thing in mind besides food, music, movies, and books. But that one thing just happened to be a gaping abyss in my life. Simone offered up a platter and I eagerly stepped on to be the appetizer and the dessert of this lunch date.

We had a good time together. He made me laugh often, and how desperately I needed that! He played cuts from the extensive collection of music CD's stacked in Tower of Pisa fashion around his stereo. He filled my mind, so I didn't think beyond food, music and the narcotic of lovemaking. I was thirsty for the touch of a man and bewitched by intense desire. For a few hours, the pain subsided.

Simone's idea of a perfect afternoon was to make love and then cook, sitting me down with a glass of wine while he chopped garlic and rosemary or splashed lemon sauce over chicken or mixed up a simple but tastebud-tweaking pasta. Our meals ended with an espresso made in the ever-present Italian stovetop coffee maker. I'd help tidy up and then he'd drive me back to the center of town with the excuse of an important appointment he had to run off to.

We had several such afternoons while I was in Florence, but in the end, in spite of a glimmer of deeper connection, Simone and his Tuscan delights failed as a band-aid. I was lonelier than before I arrived. When he went off to Naples on business, I found myself alone again in Florence. Wandering aimlessly through the streets, I crossed a bridge over to the *altr'arno*, the other side of the Arno river, came upon the Renaissance church of Chiesa Santo Spirito, and stepped inside. Years of grief spilled out.

Chapter Eighteen
The Dawning

What lies behind you
And what lies in front of you
Pales in comparison
To what lies inside of you

- Ralph Waldo Emerson

S imone and I continue emailing several times a week after my return to Bali. We aren't the answer for each other, but this Florentine dalliance has served a purpose, giving each of us hope and distraction when life is almost unbearable. He isn't a replacement for the deep relationship that I've lost with Bob and I'm not the love of his life, but our liaison has been a temporary oasis for us both.

After the agony in Italy, I want to do something with the experience besides just tuck it away in my memory. I wonder if it could be helpful to other caregivers. They must have confusing deep grieving issues as well.

The idea sprouts for an article, 'Grieving The Loss of a Loved One to Alzheimer's'. I have no idea where to publish it, but I feel driven to write it. Tens of thousands of words later,

I discover I'm writing a book, *Piece by Piece*. I don't know where it will go. I only know I have to write it because it helps me remember who my soulmate used to be and the glorious gift of love and adventure we shared. As I write, buried memories dance in my mind. Gratitude erupts.

I return to Bali with a recurring need to try to understand and define the relationship between loneliness and grief. They're tangled together in an infinite knot centered in my chest. I can abide grief, but for some reason I feel like a failure if I admit to loneliness. Even when I'm with friends, I can still feel both these emotions at the same time. That stymies me.

Does grief bring up the memories of how good Bob and I were together, and thus bring on loneliness? And why is there this pressing need to define the sadness, to categorize it? I prefer not to numb out, but to be present with it until I just can't bear it any longer. I'm flailing. Ramesh called this the flip-flop. He told us it was normal, after taking his concepts in deeply, to backslide to our old ways of being, especially when we're pushed to our emotional limits. Sometimes I feel abandoned by the teachings that buoyed me up. That leaves me even lonelier.

And living in Bali doesn't come with an Alzheimer's support group. I wonder, *Do other caregivers of spouses experience this loneliness? How do they cope?* Occasionally, I surf the Internet looking for online groups, but I'm too pressed with the nuts and bolts of everyday living to linger long on the Web.

***

Four months after the flood of tears in Chiesa Santo Spirito, I'm back in the States to do my annual Tucson shows. Heiner helps me again, as he has since Bob's bout of encephalitis. Nano and Ketut take care of Bob in our Bali house. I get email reports: 'Bob's fine. We keep adding to our bag of tricks to keep him happy. Don't worry, Susan. We can take care of him.' They attach a photo of Bob picking up leaves in the garden.

This is my longest trip leaving Bob in their care and I'm seventy-five per cent at ease, but I still sleep with my phone on in case some crisis crops up. As long as I'm focused on my work there's no time to feel the grief, and that's a relief. It's a busy six weeks, leaving me little time to myself.

Just after the shows, I drive up to Nevada City to see my accountant and eye doctor, and return things to storage until the show next year. I'm looking forward to the drive, to having Andrea Bocelli booming on the stereo and being alone in the cocoon of the van, but not more than twenty minutes into the trip, sadness highjacks me. I'm confounded that the grief is still hanging out just under the surface, waiting for a moment of silence to come to the foreground.

All the tears shed in Italy and since don't seem to have made a dent in this mountain of emotion. I feel cheated of my music and this time on my own. *When will this end?* I ask myself. *Do I have to wait for Bob to die for this sadness to be finished?* I try to remind myself to be grateful for the deep, close relationship we had, and for having been so well loved. But try as I might, this brings little consolation.

I'm flip-flopping now from the excitement of loving what

I'm doing to this heaviness of heart. I know acceptance is the only possibility for healing. But I can't seem to find it.

***

Bob does well for the ten weeks I'm in the States. Whenever he asks, Nano and Ketut tell him I'm on a visa run and will be back in a few days. In Bob's mind, as long as I'm doing something necessary and will return soon, he's satisfied. Hanna and Keith have taught us that using the same answer repeatedly gives someone with Alzheimer's a feeling of familiarity and safety, so even though we want to be creative with our answers, we stick to the well-worn oldies.

I'm comforted that the carers are doing so well, and that Bob is safe and healthy, but my return to Bali brings little peace. I continue to feel displaced, as though there's no room for me in this home since Bob wants it closed up tight once evening arrives and it becomes unbearably hot and stuffy. I feel I have nowhere to go for comfort. I have a difficult time focusing; my mind is abuzz with what needs to be done.

While I was away in Tuscon, the staff decided how to care for Bob - what he would eat and where to take him for excursions - but now that I'm back everyone looks to me to make the decisions. Wayan wants to know what to cook. Nano and Ketut want to know what hours to work. I watch my energy leak through the cracks of the day. I can't quite grab hold of life - it feels like I'm viewing it from a distance.

Five weeks after my return, I'm sitting in our lush, tropical garden lost in the beauty of the sun glinting off rain-splashed leaves. Nano has taken Bob for a ride, giving me time to myself, and I'm crying.

Loneliness, burn out, grief – where's the joy? Where's the wonder of this garden? I have magic smack dab in front of me, but I can't feel it. Where's my 'can do' attitude? Where's the light?

When I look at a website on caregiver burn-out, I convince myself I don't have it because it feels like failure to admit to it. When I think how fortunate I am to have patient, affordable caregivers while many in the West have to care for a loved one with Alzheimer's on their own, when I consider that I live in a tropical paradise and have work that I love, I feel more pathetic and more like a failure. This is my reality. I so want to embrace and accept it, but I can't seem to accomplish that. I'm short with everyone - employees, friends, Bob, myself. Every little thing sets me off. I can't seem to find a place of comfort, inside or out.

Bob's ability to communicate is doing a nosedive. He struggles to find elusive words, using 'thing' as a substitute for nouns, and makes no sense at times. He asks for the thing to stir his tea or the white stuff to sprinkle with the thing.

One afternoon he asks me, "When are we leaving this place?"

I tell him calmly, "It's our home."

"Well, I might not want to live here anymore," he says in a cranky tone. His eyes are dark and gloomy. He's fidgeting and can't seem to sit still.

"But my work is here!" I croak, trying not to react outwardly, but feeling desperate inside.

"Then I might not want to live with you anymore if you want to stay here," he says, like a child trying to get its way.

Even though I know this is the disease speaking and not my husband, I feel slapped. Once again I'm shedding weight and my friends are worried. I'm not sleeping well. *How much longer can you do this, Susan?* I ask myself.

By June 2010 I'm planning another escape to Italy. This time I want to formally study Italian and see other places besides Florence. I want to be anywhere but home.

***

Finally, after months of ineffective attempts to stop the leaks in my sleeping cabin, I hire a new contractor who strips the roof completely off, installs rubber sheeting over the plywood and moves the tiles closer together. I sleep at Cat's house for the week it takes to finish the job. At last, the cabin is secured against the elements. The new roof and Italy plans give me hope and a modicum of inner peace. In spite of Bob's ongoing incontinence and items going missing, I'm less irritable.

Then Made, our office manager, leaves a thousand dollars on the computer table while he uses the bathroom before going to town to change the money into local currency. When he comes out of the bathroom, the money is gone. This reliable and honest man is beside himself. Five of us search the house in a panic. Bob, of course, can't remember seeing it. Finally, after twenty minutes of looking, I pick up a box of tissues and there it is. Bob hid it to protect us, just as he does the computer mouse and whatever else he perceives is of value. Made bursts into tears. The Balinese rarely show their emotions publically, and to see this polite, dignified man reduced to this embarrassing state undoes me.

Margie points out, "You have a few good days and you think you can continue to do this. Then Whack! It all goes to hell. You're burned out, Susan. It's time to face up to that."

I start to hear rumblings from friends and neighbors that my staff are reaching breaking point, and if I don't want to lose them, I'll have to find a solution. I don't have the money to move the whole office and workshop. When we have an employee meeting, they inform me that I'm so stressed I'm not dealing with either them or Bob in a helpful manner. I'm crying so often they're afraid to talk to me.

I've come face to face with the searing wall of burn-out, and the consequence of that is unbearable: I have to find an alternate place for Bob to live. The only choice I can see is an Alzheimer's unit in the States because there are no such facilities on Bali.

I go the gym to work off some of the anxiety and run into an old acquaintance whom I haven't seen for ages. He tells me what happened to both his parents in nursing homes: abuse and over-drugging. "My sister is suing one of the facilities as we speak," he tells me. My heart pounds and acid pours into my stomach. How can I leave Bob in one of those places? We don't have money for a state-of-the-art facility. I'd have to put him where the State dictates. What's best for him? For us?

I feel backed against a wall. "No matter what I do, it'll be a lose-lose situation," I tell Margie. "If I leave Bob somewhere, it'll be like cutting off my arm and abandoning it. If I try to continue caring for him at home, I risk losing our business and my sanity. He needs to be safe. He needs full-time care and a stimulating environment. And exercise. How can I ensure that if I have to rely on the government? I feel I'd be sending him to the dog pound."

I leave for Bangkok and Italy knowing that when I return I'll have to make a decision. I want to put it off as long as I can. I want to bury my head so far in the sand it comes out the other side into a pain-free Shangri-la.

***

I'm sitting at Vivi, my favorite Bangkok coffee shop on the edge of the Chao Praya River. A sense of wonder stirs in me as the first orange shafts of sunset mix with the water's reflections. Then the wonder becomes tinged with trepidation about the decision looming five weeks ahead of me. In my head, I hear myself telling friends, "I can't live like this anymore. I'm looking into placing Bob." But inside I don't really believe I'll do it. I keep hoping for a miracle, a way to keep Bob in Bali – something no one has thought of yet. I need divine guidance, divine intervention. When I'm able to stay present, the trepidation is replaced by the excitement of travel and a sense of renewal from being out of the Alz grind. I'm less sad, less grief-stricken, and less lonely when I don't think about what faces me when I return to Bali.

Before I leave Bangkok for the flight to Milan, I receive an email that Bob slipped out of the house and away from Ketut and was found wandering the streets of Ubud confused and lost. A friend who didn't know he has Alzheimer's found him. Shocked by the change in Bob since she'd last seen him, she led him home. I pray I won't be called home by a disaster before this respite trip is over.

I board the plane for Italy armed with Lauren Kessler's *Finding Life in the Land of Alzheimer's*, a book about working at a state-of-the-art Alzheimer's care facility. I hope it'll bring me closer to finding peace if I decide to place Bob in America.

In the old part of Verona, I treat myself to a cozy room with a burgundy-red frescoed ceiling and ancient arches that transport me to another era. While it's over my budget, I don't have the heart to travel on the cheap right now. I tell myself, "You won't miss this money in six months."

Wandering the winding streets with little traffic, I explore for hours. Lured by a bountiful display in a fruit store on a narrow twisting lane, I buy a perfectly ripe peach and five apricots. These are two of the few things that I miss in Bali. I eat them on the street, their juice running down my hand, their perfume delighting my senses.

Eventually, I come upon the Roman Arena, where operas are performed nightly. A stage set surrounds the two thousand year old building: Madame Butterfly's tall Chinese street lanterns, dragons, and curlicue roof decorations flank the exposed masonry of the arena. Joy peaks out for the first time in ages as I'm awed by this juxtaposition and overtaken by photo possibilities. Zooming in, cutting off defining elements, and making abstract expressions of this visual extravaganza, I'm almost dancing with my camera. On the opposite side of the arena are the sets for the Verdi opera, Aida, with a menagerie of sphinxes and Egyptian animal gods all painted with gold and rainbow colors. This is heaven.

Within a few days, my tortured Italian gets easier to dredge up out of the tangled depths of my mind. I even start dreaming in it. I'm having fun and the Italians encourage me.

My back and shoulders relax as I realize my stress level has bottomed out. I put salt in my coffee, the train to Modena is delayed, and I shrug these problems off and order another coffee, happy to be where I am. Happy. It's been so long that I'd forgotten what it's like to be easy with life instead of fighting impossible daily battles. I wonder, *Is it possible to be in the middle of stress and go with it instead of fighting it?* Maybe years of mediation are paying off.

Greg, a Bali friend, has sent me to his family in Modena. Normally I'd be too shy to visit people I don't know, but something urges me to go. I'm writing in my journal, waiting for Greg's cousin to pick me up at the train station. He's late, but again I'm happy to just be where I am. I look up to see a tall, thin, gray-haired man standing over me.

Giuliano has easily picked me out from the other patrons. We joke about my numerous heavy bags. He deftly packs them into his old car, which he apologizes for. It makes me smile to see the floors littered with detritus. No pretentions here, just a down to earth kind of guy. He tells me that if I don't like his friend's apartment, where he's arranged for me to stay, that he'll take me to a hotel, but when I see it, I feel comfortable in the simply furnished fourth floor walk-up. And it helps that it's inexpensive since I went over budget in Verona. The church bells clang, my heart swells. I'm here in Italy and I feel I'm floating, weightless.

Giuliano calls me later in the day and invites me to a book launch and dinner. Our walk to the event becomes part city tour. He points out the Luciano Pavoratti Theater, where he works as second in command of lighting. We pass the Duomo, a Romanesque cathedral built in the 1100's, now a World Heritage Site. He leads me in to see its famous Rosetta window, which is casting a light show on the adjacent wall. Giuliano is passionate about light and lighting; he tells me that, as the light travels across the wall during the day, it rarely looks the same twice.

Out on the street he shows me things I'd have never seen on my own. "Look up," he says. I follow his finger to see an ancient stone shell, a symbol of protection, inset into the corner of a pillar. He's a walking guidebook full of facts and figures about his city.

After the launch we walk to dinner, talking the entire time. When Guiliano isn't pointing out the sites, he tells me about his life, about his dashed ambitions to be an archeologist and his love of Sumerian art. He confides that after a couple of stressful years taking care of his aging parents, he lost his father. His mother is frail after recent intestinal surgery. He needs a break and is planning a trip to Bali to see Greg, arriving the same time that I return.

I tell him about Bob and the decision I'm facing, and how Italy is a respite trip for me. He knows little about Alzheimer's but he understands what it's like to be a caregiver. We eat Napolitano pizza, the best I've ever had, brimming with squid, muscles, clams in their shells, shrimp, and cockles, all on a delightfully thin crust with no cheese. He drizzles olive oil over the pie and we dig in. When we exhaust ourselves, he walks me back to my room and politely says goodnight.

The next day I'm invited to lunch in the centuries old palazzo where his family lives. Giuliano's mother and his aunt, both octogenarians, greet me warmly. Cousin Marco arrives for lunch and the small white family dog dances welcome around everyone's feet. We sit down to paper-thin slices of veal accompanied by a Russian salad.

Guilano pours ice cold Prosecco into flutes as the dishes are passed round amid a vivid political conversation. I try to keep up but finally sit back watching the flying hands of Italian communication. I'm over my head in understanding, but I'm so enjoying being here. There are roasted green beans and onions, bitter leaves of raddicio and a savory tart with tomatoes and olives. Food in Italy is almost a national religion. When a fruit bowl brimming with peaches, nectarines and cherries is passed, I choose perfectly ripe, juicy cherries – a fruit I haven't eaten in years. And as if that isn't enough, an apricot tart and the cookies I've brought are served with espresso.

Giuliano is one of those people I feel I've known in some other 'before'. Over the next three days, we marathon talk the afternoons into the wee hours propped up on his couch with pillows, stroking Olmo, his ginger cat. Sipping tea as we talk, he opens up, revealing things he's rarely exposed to others, including details about the recent end of a fifteen-year relationship. He's clear he doesn't want another one. "I never want a woman to control my feelings again," he says bitterly.

He studies my photography and paintings, intently taking more time than anyone else ever has, carefully studying each piece. He asks, "How do you get the ideas for the paintings?"

"I either see the image or it's described in my head. Sometimes, it arrives complete. Sometimes, I start a piece and then more instruction comes to me."

Through our mutual opening I feel he really understands my creativity and from where it stems. We both feel understood, and this deep connection transports us away from life's serrated edges. I've found the connection I've been craving, but without the physical intimacy that seals it into a third being – an 'us'.

We laugh a lot. His broken English and my fractured Italian is fodder for our humor. We are talking about one of his favorite subjects, music, and he states more than asks, "You know Loraid?"

"No," I say, hesitating, feeling a bit stupid.

"You don't know Loraid?" he says incredulously. Then he starts singing *Walk on the Wild Side* and says, "You really don't know? How can you not know Loraid?" Finally it dawns on me he means Lou Reed and I double over in stitches, tears streaming down my face. This is part of what I need – to be silly, to laugh, to be myself.

While Giuliano works at the theater during the day, I explore Modena, an elegant city with grand, colorful palazzos flanking wide avenues, and smaller streets branching off. The city feels tall, as if it's reaching for the sky. It makes me want to stand up straight.

I wander, photographing the city, until I find the fresh market. There are figs, nectarines, strawberries, raspberries, and blackberries. The array of cheeses, olives and prepared foods such as marinated eggplant with capers or tiny tomatoes tossed with fresh buffalo mozzarella has me clicking away.

I catch my breath in a pew in the Duomo, soaking up the silence forged from centuries of devotion. I walk softly in that sacred space, melting into the energy. The womb-like crypt with it's many-arched ceiling and multi-colored marble pillars stills my mind. An ancient pulpit begs to be caressed, the cool stone housing the secrets of thousands of hands, the balustrade worn smooth from eons of touch. I'm content. This is the trip I'd longed for last year when I'd melted into a puddle of tears, broadsided by grief and loneliness. To feel these old friends return - joy, wonder, the creative spark - makes my heart soar. I feel resurrected, at least for now.

**

I move on to Florence, where a tiny apartment with a cupboard-sized kitchen becomes my home for three weeks. Its frescoed ceiling greets me morning and night, continuing my sense of being a voyeur into another era. I plan to work on 'Piece by Piece' when I'm not at my Italian course or doing my homework.

Simone once again fills part of the void left by Alz, whipping up his Tuscan specialties followed by long lovemaking. But although I want to be his friend, and to feel as confident with him as I am with Giuliano, he won't let me in. It's just sex for him. It's clear he's not relationship material.

I joke to Margie in a phone call, "I have this intimate connection with Giuliano, but nothing physical, and a physical connection with Simone that's completely superficial. Maybe one day both parts will arrive in the same package!" Still, I am so grateful to both these men. They make the unbearable bearable and block out the decision looming over me.

Giuliano invites me up to Modena for a weekend gathering of friends he's known since adolescence who have stayed in touch all these years. They're a jovial group, easy with each other, and I feel instantly at ease, torturing everyone with my tattered Italian, which leads to lots of laughter. Lunch is a banquet of grilled meats and chicken, salads, and French fries, rich desserts, liquor and coffee. We talk over one another, hands flying, laughing in an Italian cacophony. Eventually, I sit back peacefully, not even trying to understand the din, but once again totally happy to be in this genial atmosphere with ten Italians bouncing jokes off one another. It doesn't matter that I miss most of them.

Giuliano and I talk the hour's drive back to town and then on into his house until one in the morning, sharing our hopes and dreams. I wonder how we can have so much to say to each other. And then the sadness comes crawling back through my happiness, turning it inside out. I keep this to myself, not wanting to break our connection.

Back in Florence and back at the language school, my days are filled to overflowing, which helps to fend off grief, but as soon as I have an empty space, it's there just under the surface. I'm growing weary of it. *Why can't I just move on?* I start to worry that my supportive friends will become impatient with me.

The closer going home approaches, the more frequently sadness spreads its cloak. It doesn't take much for tears to come. I'm certain I just have to be with it and let it be, but the urge to call someone, to go out, to do anything to avoid it, looms large.

I've been delving into Kessler's book throughout my journey; I finish it in Florence. It's a well-written insight into Alzheimer's care - what life is like for the patients in a facility and what it's like for the caregivers – and it's had me laughing, crying and cringing all at the same time. Kessler understands the people she cares for, but she's exhausted doing it. The facility where she works doesn't use drugs to control the patients. The staff use techniques, which are far better for the patients, but take time and patience.

Yet, even though Kessler is working in a top of the line Alzheimer's unit, the caregivers are only paid minimum wage. They're expected to toilet and shower the residents, help with dressing, change diapers, do laundry, empty commodes, vacuum, dust, disinfect and take out the garbage. In addition, they have to get their residents to and from activities, deal with family and friends, and fill out a detailed daily logbook about their shift. Then, in their 'spare' time, they're expected to interact thoughtfully and compassionately with the residents. The low pay and demanding work mean most staff only stay a maximum of a year. Yet people with Alzheimer's have a hard time with change. They need the stability of reliable people with whom they're familiar.

Instead of the solace I'd hoped for, Kessler's words bring me distress. The unit she works in is a corporation and they don't value the activity director who brings music, animals to pet, art and entertainment for the residents. Their bottom line is profit, not making the residents content. How can I send Bob to America to live in one of these places? How would I even get him there? And he's a physical man; he needs freedom to garden and exercise. The thought of sending him away twists my stomach into a deep ache. Yet I'm burned out. I feel like a traitor. Even if I could afford a place with good care, I still wish there was a way to keep him in Bali. I stop working on 'Piece by Piece' because the writing is bringing up everything I need respite from.

My office manager, Made, emails, "Bob has been very calm the last four days. He even brought me water and salt when I ate lunch at the office. It made me want to cry." Denial whispers, "Maybe the situation's not so bad after all." As strange as it seems, I keep getting waylaid by denial, perhaps as a protection from the decision that's looming and that I don't want to make. The decline rate of the disease is not linear and neither are my emotions.

I spend my last day in Florence shopping for gifts and packing. Simone calls to have a last coffee. We enjoy the time together, laughing, and talking – he always points out bits of Florence that only Florentines know. After a few kisses, Simone is off. I feel our relationship has fulfilled its purpose and is complete. It's time for me to move on. Food and sex only carry my interest so far. I need depth and connection. Yet when I think of him, gratitude wells up for appearing when he did. He's been a beacon of possibilities, lighting the way through two of the hardest years in Alz World.

I walk away, saying goodbye to the city. The light is theatrical, the buildings grand, and I feel I'm seeing Florence through fresh eyes. I end up at Rivoli in Piazza Signorina for a last people-watching with a Spritz Aperol, remembering how often Bob and I came here when we were in Florence the year he came to Filicudi to claim me. I have a front row table, just as we did, with the same clear view of Palazzo Vecchio, David, Neptune, and all the tourists snapping memories.

Winding down, going home to face the inevitable, I take the train to Modena for one more evening with Giuliano and find I've left my overflowing cosmetic bag in the apartment back in Florence. In Bangkok, I get severe food poisoning and have to be wheelchaired to a bathroom and then to the taxi stand. The clincher is missing my flight home to Bali by one day. I'm a seasoned traveler, yet somehow I miss the fact that a day is lost flying from Milan to Bangkok. Miraculously, I'm given a stand-by seat on the very full airplane. Is this resistance or what?

Chapter Nineteen
Never Never Land

We cannot find the way to Peace
Peace is the Way.
We cannot find the way to Joy
Joy is the way.

- A. J. Muste

B ob is all smiles when I walk through the gate. He hugs me hard. For a moment, swept up in his embrace, I think, *This isn't so bad*. Five minutes later he's forgotten that I've just returned. Alz World sucks me back in. As the afternoon wears into evening, I undergo a refresher course in living with a deconstructing spouse.

The next day Nano and Ketut and my business staff catch me up on Bob's shenanigans: his walkabouts, on and off incontinence, food obsessions, irritations, his packing and hiding things. Nothing has changed. It's still clear that I need to separate Bob from the business or I stand to lose my dedicated employees.

The staff at Siam Sally's welcome me and indicate Cat is already upstairs. I'm excited to see my dear friend for a catch-up on Ubud life and a debriefing from my trip. She's sitting at a round table near a window with a tall, frozen lychee martini already in front of her. I quickly order the same.

"So, tell me about your trip - I'm dying to hear!"

I give her a detailed description, including Simone, Giuliano, the language school, the food I ate and learned to cook, and the places I explored. "It was everything I hoped last year would be. It was a new world while I was there." I take a deep breath. "But the problem with going away is that everything lays in wait for my return. Yes, I had five glorious weeks. But now I'm back in the mire and it feels like I never went anywhere."

"Did you decide what to do about Bob?"

"I've agonized over this, Cat." I slump down in my chair. "I know I can't keep him at home anymore. But it tears my heart out to think of moving him back to the States and leaving him there. Yet I have to be here to run the business." My voice quivers. "We need the business to eat." Cat watches me with eyes that indicate she's processing something as I speak. "I need divine intervention, Cat. I need a whole new way to look at this."

Cat's quiet for a few moments, tapping her cheek with her forefinger. Then she says cautiously, "I just finished helping my gardener and his wife renovate a small cottage next to their family compound. I pictured it perfect for a single woman who wants to be in a quiet village close to Ubud." She takes a sip of her drink before she says, "But it could be suitable for Bob."

I used to envision my sleeping cabin as a place to house Bob when he became wheelchair bound in some distant future.

Before burnout, it hadn't occurred to me that I'd get to the point of not being able to live with him before that time came, so I'd only superficially considered a different Bali house for him. I was so overwhelmed with work, caregiving and grieving, that the idea of having to search for a house, set it up, and find more caregivers was daunting. I just couldn't take any more on. Once burnout occurred, it was as though my mind had gotten stuck in a groove, thinking I'd have to take him back to America. While I desperately didn't want to do that, it seemed the only alternative. So the idea of a place available now where Ketut and Nano could continue to care for him makes me sit up and lean in. "When can I see it?"

"Tomorrow, if you like."

"Tomorrow it is!"

"If you take it, I'll throw in my dachshund, Daisy. She isn't happy in my multi-dog household. She starts quarrels with the other two."

"That would be perfect! Bob grew up with dachshunds." Thinking of Daisy living with Bob triggers a memory from our Sri Lanka trip. We were walking on a beach when we were approached by a man who had cabins for rent. Feeling tired, Bob plopped down on the white sand while I checked out the cabins. When I returned, there he was sitting cross-legged with his arm draped around a large, light brown dog that was sitting up as close to him as possible. The memory makes my heart smile.

"Do you know the cost of the cottage?"

"About $250 dollars a month."

"I can afford that!"

We toast to divine intervention and martini-inspired ideas. And dogs.

Driving home, my heart pounds with excitement as I wonder if this will really work. I don't want to anger Bob or make him more anxious, and I especially don't want him to feel I'm abandoning him. I know he still retains emotions even if memories are elusive. But I've held out for so long, thinking I could keep him at home, that it's both exhilarating and terrifying to think that a suitable, separate place might be imminently possible.

Back at home I pull Ketut aside to tell him about this new idea. I ask if he and Nano can make it work since Bob needs twenty-four hour care and they need their family life.

"I have a friend who wants to learn to work with Bob. He has no experience, but he's very patient. I think we can train him. Then we'll need just one more man." Excitement mixes with relief as I realize Ketut is way ahead of me.

The next morning I meet Nano and Ketut in Singakerta, a quiet village ten minutes from Ubud, to see if they think Cat's gardener's house might work. The small blue cottage sits off a quiet lane next to a *warung*, an open-air shop selling tea, coffee, sachets of shampoo and other necessities. The house has one bedroom, a sitting room, a bathroom, a kitchen, and a veranda with a sofa and dining table. We'd have to get a sofa bed for the night caregiver and a TV and DVD player for entertainment. We learn the small garden will soon be expanded so Bob would have plenty of space for gardening.

I tally the costs. I'd need about $24,000 a year for the house, four caregivers, and other expenses. I don't have it. But I'm determined to find a way to earn the extra cash. We'll have to share our sixteen-year-old car since I can't afford another one. That'll be a challenge. *But it just might work!* I try not to get my hopes up too high for fear they'll be dashed.

The boys agree to give it a try for a few months. They know they'll be on twelve-hour shifts, with little time for personal life, but that'll motivate them to look for another man to train.

A friend suggests that I see if the Veteran's Administration will help with Bob's costs since he was on active duty during the Korean War. I had no idea that there was even a remote possibility of financial assistance, but after Bob's daughters look into it, the VA man says we have a good chance of help. We start the process of gathering discharge papers, doctor's reviews, marriage and divorce certificates, tax returns, caregiver duties, and expenses.

On September 1, 2010, I pay the first month's rent on the Bob House. I can't believe I'm doing this. I never thought I'd have the courage to make this decision. Both our doctor in Bangkok and the Alz angels, Hanna and Keith, confirm that I'm doing the right thing. "It's time," they all agree.

I've learned from Internet research, books, and Keith and Hanna, that caregivers often wait too long, hoping it won't come to this. It usually takes burnout or a dramatic turn of events such as their own ill health to force them to make the decision. I hope I haven't waited too long. I feel emotionally tattered, walking the razor's edge of sanity as I start surreptitiously packing Bob's things and planning the move.

For the next week, Ketut or Nano takes Bob to the new house to play with Daisy, who's transported there each day in a basket on a motorbike, her ears flying and a doggie smile on her face. They start with less than an hour, working up to several hours a day. Wayan, our cook, brings Bob's lunch that she's prepared at home. He naps and gardens, believing he's visiting Ketut's house, and seems comfortable having familiar faces around him.

My staff shift into full gear making lists of what we need to do to make the move as stress free as possible for all of us, but especially for Bob. Still, I'm awash with tears when they go home each day.

On the morning of the move, I walk into the house from my sleeping cabin to a pile of wet sheets on the floor. Bob has peed in the bed, something that hasn't happened since before I left for Italy. He must be picking up on my anxiety. And now I'm crying again. I need the intensity to stop.

Nano and Ketut take Bob to the beach, promising not to return for five hours. Our staff and I focus, packing what's left and moving everything to the little blue house. We put up familiar pictures, neatly stack some of Bob's clothes on shelves and hang up others. The new TV and DVD player are set up and we create a cozy, comfortable environment, plumping pillows and placing flowers in vases. Everyone is working hard to pull this off, hoping that Bob will make this transition in peace. We leave before he and the boys arrive.

The Alz Angels have advised me not to see my husband for

two weeks, and then to see him on neutral territory. "It's best not to bring him back to your house," they've told me. Although I understand the need for this, it feels cruel to both of us.

I come home weary, guilty, and sad, to find a three-foot long monitor lizard wreacking havoc in the kitchen as it tries to find a way out. After a crash bang chase over the stove and behind the fridge, the staff capture him with a fish net and take him outside. We set to work cleaning up the mess and I slowly start to reorganize the house since we've taken some furniture to Bob's and emptied shelves we shared. I don't want to do too much in case he has to come back.

Once the staff are gone, I roam the house. I'm too apprehensive to enjoy the peace. This is like death or divorce. I'm nauseous and headachy. I want to crawl out of my skin and feel faint from the intensity. My throat closes. I thought death would take one of us. I never expected to lose Bob piece by excruciating piece. I never thought we'd live apart.

Later, Ketut calls to tell me that they had a pleasant outing, with Bob napping on the drive home. But when they walked into the cottage, Bob roared, "What are my things doing here?" Ketut tried to appease Bob by telling him that his house is being renovated and no one can live there while the roof is taken off. When Bob demanded to know where I was, Ketut told him I was on a visa run in Bangkok, but would join him in a few days. Bob grumped and complained, but soon settled down for the evening.

***

Several days later, Ketut tells me that it's taken Bob a few nights to get used to the different noises at his new house and sleep well, but that he's adapting. I feel a tentative relief, but am too much on edge to let myself sink into it. Then I find out the toilet leaks, the shower only has hot water and the windows need curtains. I try to sort these issues out without going to the cottage until the two-week quarantine period is up. Meanwhile, it's a challenge sharing the car, and Wayan slam bangs around the kitchen, stressed by needing to have all Bob's daily food ready by eleven each morning for his carers to pick up. This new program will take getting used to for all of us.

At least Asa, the new man in training, is doing well. While he's timid, has minimal English and doesn't drive a car, he and Bob seem to find common ground. And he's patient. But we still need a fourth caregiver.

We start to interview. Many want the decent salary earned working with a foreigner, but it's a rare man who can cope with Bob's mental state. If he were physically incapacitated, they would have no problem, but having to tell fibs to redirect him is beyond their comprehension. Finally, Krok, a man from Ketut's village, comes forward. He drives, speaks passable English, and is motivated to learn. He starts training immediately.

Three weeks after Bob moves, a magical moment lightens my heaviness when a velvety black dragonfly buzzes around the kitchen, looking for a way out. I observe him for a while, and then say out loud, "Come on! Let's go outside." He lands on my outstretched thumb and we walk out into the garden. In the sunlight, he transforms into a stained glass window. His black wings have transparent olive green at the top and tiny magenta windows inset into the black while his body has mosaic patches of robin's egg blue with a red dot behind his head. He stays until we have our fill of each other and then off he flies.

I'm transported back to Filicudi and the dragonfly who came to be sketched for my painting twenty-six years earlier. Warmth fills my chest. Moments like this are candles in the dark cave I seem to be residing in. They give me a glimmer of hope that I won't always feel so cut off from joy.

Gradually, I make changes at home – adding garden lights, freshening up the paint on the veranda, and getting a new couch cover made. I've been afraid to enjoy the house for fear this experiment will fail, but I'm finally allowing myself to breathe a bit easier. I'm reclaiming this home from which I'd disengaged, letting Bob have it whatever way made him less anxious. Now there's no more TV droning on, no sauna-like living room, no urine odor. I have my own towel and know my toothbrush won't be used to clean anything but my teeth.

Still, I'm fragile. Sitting at the dining table trying to choke back tears and choke down food, Bob's empty place torments me with loneliness. The Angels and the caregivers are encouraging me not to see him too often, not to overdo it for both our sakes.

***

For our first date after the move, I settle in at Tutmak's, a café we've often frequented. I arrive before Bob because he has little patience for waiting.

"It's great to see you!" Bob says as he hugs me. "We're so lucky to have this life, to travel the world together. It's great to be back here!" He looks around the restaurant and out at the adjacent soccer field. "I love this place." He thinks he's been away, but I can tell he's not sure where he is.

"Text us when you're ready to go," Nano and Ketut request as they go back to the car, leaving us alone.

We chat about this and that, with me steering the conversation towards Bob's interests. I notice his long-term memories are splintering. His mind is stringing fragments from various memories together to create a whole new scenario that makes sense to him, but which I know isn't accurate. When he veers off, I follow, trying to adjust my perspective quickly to reinforce wherever he is, pretending I know exactly what he's talking about.

Before we order dessert, Bob goes through his pockets, emptying them on the table. He looks at every item as though it's the first time he's seen it, then puts it all back. I can see he's gradually becoming more anxious. A few minutes later he repeats the process.

"I don't have a cent on me!" he exclaims.

"I'm treating you to dinner tonight, Honey. You probably left your money on the dresser."

"How could I go out without a dime?"

"No worries, you have a rich wife," I tease him. "Besides, it's my turn to pay". I kiss his cheek.

After a walk around town and back to the car, parting is difficult.

"Bob, I have an appointment with Margie. We're working on

a website. We have a deadline." I know he won't be interested in joining anything to do with a computer.

"When will I see you?" He's hanging on to me as I try to encourage him to get in the car.

"Nano will take you home now. I'll see you there soon."

"How soon?"

"In about two hours," I say, knowing it's not true, but also knowing it'll ease his anxiety.

Finally, he's in the car. I kiss him good-by and tell him how much I love him, and off they go.

My heart sinks as I walk home. I barely get through the gate before my tears transform into sobbing. I feel I'm abandoning my love.

Yet I know this is a dream come true. Bob isn't in an institution behind locked doors. He's in his beloved Bali, with caregivers who really care about him and keep him safe. He eats and naps when he wants, works in the garden, plays badminton and goes to the gym. The caregivers take him for excursions to the beach or a swimming pool or just for a drive if the noise in the village gets too intense for him.

Our weekly dinners vary in intensity. When the veil of Alz is thick and I can't feel Bob behind it, it's easier on me. When he makes less sense, I stay more neutral. At these times he's not very affectionate. But when he's loving and sweet, it takes me days to recover because my reaction to that is instant and physical, leaving me confused.

Sometimes friends meet us for dinner, which eases the

pressure. Bob seems to enjoy that. Even though he doesn't remember the person's name, he knows they're familiar. His inhibitions have long ago lost their control valves, so the conversations can be 'interesting'.

One evening Heiner meets us at an old haunt, a restaurant called Batan Waru. When the staff welcome us by name, Bob tells the young waitress, "You're so beautiful!" His eyes are sparkling in appreciation. As the two men banter and talk, Bob comments about the slim-bottomed waitress serving the next table and pretends to grab her when she bends over. Fortunately, he doesn't make contact.

Batan Waru makes a heavenly 'Black Bottom Tart' that comes in three layers. Bob is eating the coffee mousse part when Heiner inquires, "So how is that, Bob?"

Bob looks right into Heiner's eyes and says, without missing a beat, "It's just like pussy." He hasn't lost his bawdy sense of humor.

***

As the days pass, loneliness and grief overtake me, seeming ever-present. Are these emotions more intense now because Bob is living elsewhere and they have the void that's left to do battle in? Where's the sense of relief I hoped I'd feel?

Again, I worry that my friends will become weary of me. My weight loss is turning anorexic. Secretly, I now have the body I've always wanted, but my face looks drawn and wrinkled. Is this loss of weight a way of proving what I'm going through, proving to myself how really difficult it is? Sometimes I feel I'm watching this all unfold as though it's happening to someone else.

In spite of the sadness and loneliness, I don't dwell on my husband very often. I don't miss the Bob he is now, although when I see him, I miss the Bob he was. I tell myself this is a natural part of moving into a new life. Although I'll always feel responsible for my soulmate and organize the best care I can, I tell myself I'm basically a single woman now and I'd better get used to it.

At the time, living with Helen and Lisa was the most difficult thing I'd ever had to endure. I struggled with guilt over wanting my needs met and not being able to meet theirs. I was often in turmoil, crying at the drop of a paintbrush and wondering when happiness would return. Now it feels as if I'm on a different curl of that same spiral. As I did then, I often feel numb to the intensity of what I'm living. Numbness dilutes the intensity when I bottom out, and then abates when I reach the next apex and feel alive again. The emotional tumult is staggering. It takes others observing from outside to give me a more realistic perspective.

***

I'm relying on savings to support Bob's new life, and with business down due to the current economic climate, I'm scared. It will be months until we hear from the VA. Sometimes I feel beaten down by it all and wonder where my strength and resilience have disappeared to.

These feelings build to a crescendo. Just before Christmas I have a full-blown meltdown when lukewarm coffee at breakfast pushes me over the edge. Then I find out customs has decided to return one of our standard shipments. I go ballistic.

When Margie spontaneously stops by on her way into town, it feels as though she's come to my rescue at just the right time. We settle down on the veranda couch, shoulder to shoulder, with a plate of fresh baked cream cheese brownies to dunk into mugs of hot coffee. I tell her about my meltdown. As always, she listens thoughtfully.

"Susan, this is normal. You're going through deep grief."

I start to relax as we continue to chat until she says, "I'm going for a walk with Ariana, so I won't be able to go to the gym with you today." I watch myself become jealous of the time she spends with her pregnant daughter and start to cry.

Something is very wrong. This is not about coffee, shipments, or daughters. This is about me falling apart. With the wisdom she's gained from years as a psychologist, Margie understands what's happening. She puts her arms around me and lets me cry. Finally, she says, "Come to Victoria's this afternoon. We're putting up Christmas decorations."

"I don't feel fit for human contact," I blubber.

"I won't let you stay here. You are coming!" Although I feel pathetic and try to get out of it, she persists until I agree. A few hours later Victoria greets me in a Santa hat, Linda presents me with a cup of eggnog and Margie gets us all laughing. We decorate for hours. In the end it's just what I need to pull out of the quagmire of self-pity, self-loathing, and loneliness that feels as if it will eat me.

Chapter Twenty
Rescue Puppies

It's twilight
As I walk through the garden
Turning on lights
Over the Buddha
In front of the Balinese altar
A thin coolness brushes my bare shoulders
Warm ribbons of gratitude
Stream from my heart
Countering the outer chill
I say out loud to the fish
To the flowers
To the palms
To the dragonflies
And to all things living in the garden
I say,
"Thank You!"
Thank you for this life
For light after years of darkness
Thank you for the gift of love
Friendship
Passion
Thank you!

I take to interviewing my single women friends, trying to find the key to thriving on my own, or at least being at peace with it. I need to understand this new state, and quickly.

I observe how acutely aware I am of men. I walk into a room and unconsciously take stock. At the gym, I survey who's on the treadmill, the free weights, and the elliptical. I categorize them as taken, too young, too old, gay, or possibly unattached. I didn't used to do this, but now I'm single with a husband and I feel invisible.

Ubud is filled with happy, independent woman, shakers and movers who run businesses or non-profits, who write or paint or do whatever they do man-less and fulfilled. I bore into them, asking how they do it. I hold them up to the light one by one, trying to discover their secrets. They tell me they rarely get lonely. Some don't like the way they change if they're attached to a man, some say they have no room in their lives for a relationship, and others say it would complicate their contentment. I try to convince myself, *I can do this. I just need a little help to join their ranks.*

I ask my single friends if they notice the men in a room when they enter, but most just see people. "Time will take care of the loneliness, Susan. You'll get used to being on your own," counsels Mary, who's watched Bob slowly disintegrate. I'm not convinced. I'm beginning to think something's radically wrong with me, and that I'm letting womanhood down by being so needy.

My sister assures me, "Some people are just relationship people. That's who we both are. You might as well accept it."

Eight months earlier, I'd written in my journal that I'd like a lover and I listed the qualities I'd like him to have. I completely forget this entry and on December 15, 2010 I write again in my journal:

I'd love a relationship. It would have to be with a man that's not afraid of an unconventional one where we might not be together all the time. I don't think I want another 24/7, at least not right now. The man would also have to accept that I will always love Bob and that he's my responsibility and I'll do my best for him. I'm open to someone who lives somewhere else so we have some space between us and then maybe later we evolve into living together.

I'm a relationship person. I do 'being in love' really well, as my track record proves. I just want to know that I love someone and he loves me back and we can miss each other desperately and be totally together when we are together. Plus I want to be who I am fully and not have to curb my enthusiasm!

It has to be a deep connection where we really like each other and respect each other's opinions and don't need to change each other. We are able to be open and honest even when feelings are uncomfortable.

I'd like this man to be my muse if possible or at least to understand the creative process and to honor how important it is for me.

Cat suggests I put this and any other wishes I have with my bronze statue of the Hindu God Ganesha, the Remover of Obstacles. I make another list, this one showing the hindrances I'm facing, and place the two lists inside the hollow bottom of the statue that sits on the teak dresser in my sleeping cabin. While I'm not superstitious, here in Bali this symbolic gesture feels right.

At the same time, I have a session with Janette, an Australian energy healer, because I can't find my way out of the darkness of depression. I don't easily entrust my psyche to other people, but Cat highly recommends her and I'm desperate. Whatever hocus pocus she does, I go into a deep trance for an hour and a half and come out feeling I've pushed off bottom and am headed for the light. However long it takes to reach it, at least I can see it again, up there on the surface.

***

I'm nervous about the dreaded first holiday season apart from Bob, but Margie wrangles me an invitation to a Christmas Eve party. I dress elegantly, feeling hopeful and festive for the first time in ages.

As soon as I walk in, man scanning goes automatically into action. I hardly realize it's happening. There's an interesting European man in a blue silk shirt sitting on the couch, but he puts his arm around the woman next to him. Two handsome, well-dressed men are talking to Margie and her husband, but after assessing them, I'm sure they're gay.

I know many of the people attending, so I don't have to explain my story from square one. I've grown weary of being identified with Alz. But of course, everyone wants to know how Bob is.

Before dinner I'm introduced to Alan, a sturdy, bear-like man with long white hair, a beard, and a large skin graft that takes up most of his right cheek. A scar runs from the inside top of his eyebrow and into the graft, making his right eye droop at the outside corner. The shock of how he looks takes me aback; I'd watched a movie with Margie the night before about a man who is horribly disfigured in an automobile accident and wears a mask until the end of the movie when he takes it off, shocking the audience. Meeting Alan gives me a feeling of deja vu.

Alan is Canadian and new in town. His brother and sister-in-law are close friends with Cat and asked her to take care of him while he's in Bali. He's been working in Asia and has come for the holidays.

When I learn Alan does helicopter logging in the jungles of Borneo, my judgmental mind jumps immediately into action. Living in a country that has lost the world's highest percentage of rainforest for profit, just the word 'logging' sets my thoughts on edge. I soon move off to converse with old friends, and then everyone digs into the lavish potluck banquet before we launch into a gift exchanging game that leaves us all laughing and merry.

Maite, our hostess, puts on some good old rock and roll and Margie and I pull people onto the dance floor. A small group of women are boogying by themselves, and off and on with each other. I grab the tree murderer since he's standing on his own. "Come on! Do you like to dance?"

I'm surprised and pleased when he turns out to be an excellent dancer. "You get the badge of courage for being the only man on the floor," I tell him. At one point he drops down on his knees, dancing with me from that position. When I compliment him, he brushes it off. "I just follow what you're doing." Although I step on his toes a few times, he shrugs that off too, as though it's his fault. His politeness disarms me.

I dance off after a while so I don't hog him. Alan dances with other women, obviously in his element, but we keep coming back together. Soon, everyone is wet, shirts sticking to skin in a joyous frenzy of music and movement. At one point Alan and I hold sweaty hands and do a double loop de loop. "Let's do it again so I can be near you," he says. That takes me aback. By then the party is ending and it's time to go home.

Driving home feeling more alive than I've felt in a long time, my thoughts go to Bob, who has no clue that it's Christmas Eve. Even when he was healthy he didn't care much for the holiday and especially disliked the expectation of presents. He was the kind of man who bought things for people when he saw something he knew they'd like, but having to give went against his grain. And he would have loved the dancing tonight if he could still cope with the music. We'd had to stop dancing when loud music began to confuse him and make him anxious.

The next day I bring Bob a few Christmas gifts: a new ball cap, some chocolate, and a children's book with pop-out pieces the reader can slip into slots with the name printed below. By the time he's opened the wrappers he doesn't know why I've brought the presents.

***

HAPPY NEW YEAR!!

Sandeh, my Italian teacher and friend, and I are upstairs on the second floor of her three-story house having a Campari and Prosecco on New Year's Eve. The monsoon rains are torrential, with lightning striking close by and the winds blowing right through the blinds on her open Bali-style house. While we wait for a break in the downpour, we each shuffle her Tarot deck and ask what 2011 will bring. Sandeh, a seasoned Tarot card reader, often does readings for people. For years we've both had the habit of drawing a card for the New Year. When I turn mine over, it's The Lovers.

The rain abates and we walk under neighborhood fireworks to a restaurant. Our third floor table comes with a three hundred and sixty degree view of lightning striking all around us. The air is tense and electrical; it vibrates through us as the sky lights up again and again.

After a five course Italian meal and a glass of red wine, we can't decide what to do with the rest of the evening. We start walking towards one possible venue, but meet Alan and Cat on the way. "We're going to the Michael Franti concert - come with us!" says Cat. "I have the car."

Sandeh and I look at each other quizzically. It's starting to sprinkle and the concert is outdoors on the grounds of a huge estate on the edge of town. "We can always leave if we don't like it," I say.

The warm-up band is in full swing when we arrive and a thousand people are crowding under the covered areas and spilling out onto the vast lawn. Standing under our umbrellas, Sandeh and I join the thick congregation in front of the bandstand, stopping to chat with the many friends we run into along the way. Cat nudges me towards Alan, and in a low voice commands, "Dance with him!"

I hesitate at first, remembering that it's been at least two years since Bob and I have danced together. I love to dance, but this feels like I'm crossing a line - a delicate, almost invisible, line. It feels different from the Christmas party when Margie and I were encouraging people to dance. I teeter for what seems like forever on the edge of a decision until something pushes me forward. Soon I'm dancing Mary Poppins style under my umbrella as the rain pelts down. Alan has plunged his umbrella into the wet grass, like St. George skewering the dragon. By the time Michael Franti comes on, we're soaked and my shoes are ruined, but I feel that I've broken a barrier. In the past, I would have frumped and complained about the rain; tonight I just go with it, and in letting go, I feel wild and super-alive for the first time in ages.

At midnight, fireworks explode and there's kissing and hugging all around. When Alan and I embrace, he's respectful and careful. I know Cat has told him my story.

On New Year's morning I write to my sister, Joan:

The evening felt symbolic – as though something old and outdated has been plowed under, paving the way for something new to grow. And I think I have a dance partner and friend when Alan's here. Nice guy, but I don't feel any chemistry.

***

A few days later, Alan is speaking about helicopter logging at a Rotary meeting. I want to understand his business, and perhaps alleviate my judgments, so I plan to go, but have a flat tire on the way. I walk into the meeting just as he's calling for questions at the end, giving me enough of a sense of what he does to understand that logging the rainforests is going to happen no matter what, and that helicopter logging is a sustainable technique. When Alan dashes off to a movie afterwards with only a cursory wave, I realize I'm disappointed.

The next day I receive a text message:

Sorry to rush off. And without a hug too! I owe you a big one. Movie was fantastic. Can tell you about it over tea-coffee.

Cat reminds me he's leaving in a week, and if we want to dance together again, we'd better get a move on. I tease her, "Are you matchmaking?"

"Oh no! I just know how much you like to dance."

I text Alan suggesting coffee the next afternoon, but he's already booked. Instead, we go for dinner at Laughing Buddha, a popular eatery with a tiny dance floor. We take one of the last empty wooden tables with a bench against the back wall and order *laksa*, a lemongrass and ginger scented soup with noodles, tofu, eggs, and seafood in a sour tamarind and coconut milk infusion.

The music is rock, and when our feet can't stay still a second longer, we're ready to roll. As the music takes us, we become one with it, not caring that no one else is up, not caring what others think. We barely touch our meal until the band takes a break. That's when Alan tells me, "I made a pact that if I survived cancer I'd dance as often as possible."

He tells me that, eleven years ago, when his metastasized skin cancer was still hanging on despite two rounds of chemo, his doctors told him to go home and put his affairs in order. Instead of being beaten down by the prognosis, he investigated alternative therapies. He ran through most of his savings having massive doses of intravenous vitamin C, spending time in a hyperbaric chamber, going to shamans in the Amazon rainforest to take their tonics, and taking various workshops and trainings. He also helped with palliative care for dying cancer patients as he grappled with his own disease.

He was on a fifty-five foot catamaran off the coast of Australia when he almost died. He loves the sea and boats and had been a commercial fisherman in his youth before he got into helicopters. When he thought he might not survive cancer, he and his family decided to live his dream and sail the coast of Australia. After a year and a half, his children needed to move on with their education and his wife wanted to return to Canada. But Alan's journey wasn't finished. He stayed on the boat alone.

He'd been taking a rainforest cancer treatment, a natural form of chemo, and after some time he became so weak he couldn't feed himself even though the boat was well provisioned. In physical agony, he prayed for a pain free breath.

A couple with a much smaller boat anchored in the same

cove were camping on the beach. When they hadn't seen Alan for a few days they went to investigate, and saved his life. They cooked for him and fed him until he regained his strength. They soon became fast friends and sailed together once Alan got his sea legs back. The rainforest medicine worked. His cancer miraculously went into remission as his subsequent physical checks proved.

Five years later, he had a skin and bone graft to replace his right cheek, which had been ravaged by the disease. Listening to his story, I realize this man is special. What courage! I've always had an affinity for people who persevere against all odds. Like Bob and I, they're dreamers living their dreams.

After the last song in the second set, we're soaked with sweat, riding high and beaming. Alan takes me back to where I've left my car, and in an act of chivalry, fends off an aggressive dog. We hug for a long time, then reluctantly peel ourselves apart.

The next evening I have my weekly dinner date with Bob. As is our custom, Krok and Asa drive him to our destination and I walk. It's easier this way, so they don't have to drop me at home afterwards. We tried that once and Bob escaped from the car trying to follow me.

We meet at Tutmak, our old standby. Bob beams when he sees me and gives me a long hug. I steel myself against old feelings trying to erupt. It's as painful a meeting as all the others.

The evening starts out with me helping him choose his food. He can't keep track of what's written on the menu, so I say, "You love the Green Goddess Lasagne."

"Oh, that sounds good. What's in it?"

I explain that it's vegetarian with cheese and a creamy basil sauce and comes with a salad. By the time I've finished explaining, Bob is confused and starts to read the menu again. Everything sounds good to him, but he can't remember the items above the current one he's reading.

The waitress has been cruising our table, but I've been signaling her off while I try to get Bob to make a decision. Finally, she closes in and asks if we're ready to order. She looks at Bob, who looks to me for an answer.

"Bob will have the Green Goddess Lasagna and I'll have the mixed salad with fresh grilled tuna." Bob doesn't comment or protest.

A few minutes after the order is taken, he starts in. "What's taking so long? Did they have to go to the store to get something?"

I tell him the food will be here soon and in the meantime aren't we lucky that we have each other to talk to? I tell him how much I love him and how I love our life together, trying to dismantle his anxiety. But soon he's asking again when the food will arrive.

When the food comes, I'm served first. *Damn! When will I learn to clue them into serving him first?* I should know, after all my years in Indonesia, that it's customary to serve food as it comes out rather than waiting for all a table's orders to be ready together. Bob has no sense of boundaries, and so he reaches over the table to eat forkfuls of my dinner until his arrives. Once he has his meal, he gets creative and dips his lettuce in his water and pours his tea over the lasagne. I cringe at this, but he eats it all. Old images of my handsome, once gallant husband flash through my mind. It's so sad to see him like this.

I'm glum when I walk into Bar Luna after Bob goes home. Alan and I had arranged to meet there when we heard a quartet would be playing mellow jazz. He's sitting at one of the glass-topped tables with an iced lemongrass tea and has hugs at the ready and a shoulder to cry on. I order a glass of wine.

The dance floor is even smaller than at Laughing Buddha and no one is dancing. Alan gets up and holds his hand out to me. Several people I know are there and I still feel shy to be out publically with another man in small town Ubud, a place with few secrets and lots of gossip. But another sip of wine stills my concerns. I know Alan needs to dance. I can help with that. We become the only dancers for the evening.

Since Krok and Asa still have the car, Alan drives me home on his scooter. I invite him in for tea and discover he's traveled extensively, for work as well as pleasure, spending time in Africa, Central and South America, China, New Zealand, Australia, and Southeast Asia. He's been living in and out of hotels for several years since his tumultuous thirty year marriage fell apart. He tells me he's looking for a new place to live and Bali appeals to him. It's close to Malaysia, where he's been working for the last few years, and he likes the culture here. He's quick with languages and Malaysian is almost the same as Indonesian, so he's already one step ahead of most newcomers.

He also tells me he spent his first three weeks in Ubud quietly, having sensed he needed to take more of his cancer medicine. The dose had laid him low, and he's just coming round to normal energy now. I have a momentary future flash of having to take care of another man. Maybe it's my calling in life...

Alan is so quiet and gentle in his speech that sometimes I have to lean in to hear him. This closeness pulls us together and we start hugging, ending up prone on the veranda couch, arms around one another, kissing. But I hold myself in check. I can't bring myself to let go to more. It was easy in Italy with Simone. No one knew me there. But this is my town. Here, I'm still 'SusanandBob'. Alan doesn't push. But it's clear we're both hungry for connection.

That hunger transports us to three hours of cuddling on his couch the next evening as we continue our getting to know you stories. Alan lets me know he cares, but doesn't force anything. Hunger eventually drives us off the couch to Jazz Café for dinner and our last dancing together for months. The staff know both of us, but as separate entities. They ask about Bob, adding to my self-consciousness. I see the inquisitive looks and tell Alan I need to go slowly.

But I feel the clock ticking. I'm leaving the next day for a beach weekend with Victoria and another friend, Heidi. Alan is flying to Malaysia before I get back. I'll be in the USA for two months for my annual shows when he returns to Bali. It's now or never.

"My place or yours? Or do you just want to shake hands and go our separate ways?" I can't believe I'm actually saying this as we leave Jazz Café.

"Yours. I'll go get my motor bike and meet you there."

We fall into each other's arms with a hunger that consumes

us and don't get much sleep that night. I make him leave at seven in the morning, hoping he can sneak out undetected past my landlord's house, but when my staff come in at eight-thirty with silly grins on their faces, it's obvious I've failed.

That morning I email Joan:

Please delete the email that said there is no chemistry. Alan deflowered my virgin Princess bed last night. I didn't get much sleep, but feel fantastic this morning!!

Floating to the car with Victoria and Heidi, I pass Victoria my cell phone with this message:

Today everywhere I look I see you. Every breath I take I feel you. I have no wish to complicate or clutter your life. Just know that you are well loved. Thank you so much for your time, energy, courage, and love. Have fun in Amed. Love and light, Alan

In the afternoon I receive this:

I feel your vibration in my soul, in my bones. Totally captivated I am humbled by the power of our connection. Thank you for being. My heart pounds with unbridled passion. I am on fire! Thank you thank you. Love, light, a huge hug and long searching kisses, Alan.

I'm gobsmacked. He's not only a kind, gentle man, but a poet to boot. How did I get so lucky? But we won't see each other again for nearly three months. Still, he's given me hope and recharged my empty battery.

The next morning:

Me again. Would love to spend the evening/night with you.

Could head your way and rent separate place. Back in morning for flight in afternoon. Just a thought. Missing (understatement) you. Perhaps you are enjoying the space and time away. Let me know. Love, Alan.

My heart is pounding at the prospect. "I know it's hard when a girlfriend wants to be with a man after making other plans so I don't want to cause any ill feelings between us," I tell my friends. "How would you feel if I go off with Alan to another place tonight?"

They look at each other. With a nod from Heidi, Vic says, "Why doesn't he just come here? There's plenty of room and we have tons of food." We'd made a roast turkey dinner the night before with all the trimmings, including ginger-infused mango cranberry sauce, there are plenty of leftovers, and my friends are obviously eager to meet this new man in my life.

Alan leaves Ubud on his scooter with map in hand, having never ventured far out of town on his own. It's a two and half-hour drive when you know where you're going, but there are few directional signs and often locals are of little help. Alan makes it in just over three hours. We look deeply into each other's eyes and can't keep our hands off each other, barely making it through the gate with composure. Victoria and Heidi graciously accept him into the fold, and then I lead him up to our room to drop his bag and change into swimming trunks.

The door opens onto a room with a balcony and diaphanous curtains billowing in the sea breeze. It overlooks the garden and waves beyond and has a mosquito-netted double bed, which I've decorated with a large, red flower-petal heart, with pink bougainvillea, yellow frangipani, and red hibiscus scattered in the middle. It brings him to tears. He hugs me and says, "I've never been cared for like this."

After a swim in the sea, we all gather in the kitchen to get dinner organized. With Diana Krall crooning out jazzy love tunes in the background, Alan tears basil leaves into a bowl. He's a little uneasy in this kitchen camaraderie as Heidi and Vic grill him in a friendly manner, making sure he's fit to court their friend and giving me approving looks.

It's an evening of shared stories and then it's time to take our leave. We sit on our balcony stargazing, talking, and touching to the sound of waves gently lapping the beach. It's an easy ride into deep connection, as though we've always known each other and are just reconnecting. This is what I've been craving. It's the kind of connection Bob and I shared.

It's a delicious night sleeping in each other's arms, waking, making love, sleeping again wrapped up together until sunrise when we walk along the beach as Mt. Agung glows pink in the sunrise. Alan leaves in time to pack for the airport. He lets me know he made it:

Kept the focus, made it back. Tears now too + joy and sorrow. I feel blessed. Thank you thank you for the gift of you. I feel you everywhere. I love you Susan. Life, Love and Light, Alan

I feel like Alan and I are rescue puppies brought together to love and nurture each other, and to laugh and dance with life. No problem seems unsolvable, no pain unbearable.

Bob is still my priority. I'll always love him, will always care for him to the best of my ability. But now I have someone to nurture me, to feed me in return so I can do this properly. I have so much love to give that there's plenty for both men.

Chapter Twenty-One
The Last Piece

Writing at the dining table
Out on the veranda
The last keystrokes
Tapping this book to completion
A golden dragonfly
Lands inches from my hand
With this benediction
Gratitude erupts for every joy
Every sorrow
Every challenge
On this journey of vast love

Ten months after applying to the VA for help with Bob's care, I receive the first monthly check on my sixty-fifth birthday. I can breathe easier now and take care of him without watching our meager savings evaporate. I am so grateful for this help.

When Alan is in town, he joins Bob and me on our weekly dinner dates. He also whips up beef stew, which Bob loves, when our cook has to take time off for a temple ceremony. Alan is good with Bob, bringing him out by chatting about sailing, skiing, swimming, and helicopters, all parts of Bob's life in the distant past. They joke in a male bonding way that's sometimes a bit crude and risqué. Alan accepts Bob as a big part of my life and doesn't mind appearing as only a friend when we're all together.

Bob and I are sitting down for dinner at Bolero, a new restaurant in town, when Alan walks in. I introduce him as a friend of Cat's and he pulls out a chair and shakes Bob's hand. "Cat couldn't make it tonight. She sends her apologies." While we wait for our food, Bob can't take his eyes off the old Bali photos on the café's walls. Before the Dutch insisted they cover up, it was the norm for Balinese women to be bare-breasted, and these photos are from that time.

"Wow, what a nice set!" Bob says to Alan, indicating one of the photos.

Alan agrees, but steers the conversation in another direction. "I was working on a helicopter engine the other day. Susan's told me you used to be a mech for them too."

Bob searches his mind for the memory and then mumbles something incomprehensible, smiling through his words. His attention goes back to the photos. When Alan's dinner arrives first, Bob reaches over with his fork and starts eating it. Alan good-naturedly pushes the plate closer to him so the forkfuls won't end up on the table. When it's time to leave, Alan goes first while I text the caregivers that it's time to pick up Bob.

Bob's four dedicated caregivers continue to be a Godsend, keeping him as happy and anxiety-free as possible without resorting to drugs. They work alongside him in the garden and play badminton with him in the afternoons. They take him to the gym, though he rarely works out anymore, preferring to pet the dogs that live there. They take him to the beach, the swimming pool, and for walks around the village, where the local kids sometimes accompany him. He loves this, but like a child, wants to stay and play, telling the caregivers, "You go home. I'll stay here." Their bag of tricks, gathered over the last few years, guarantees they'll get him home without a problem.

Research is finding that by letting people with dementia do what they want when they want, such as take a shower at three in the morning, walk, watch TV and eat when they want, they become less anxious and easier to manage. So if Bob gets up in the middle of the night to eat an apple or two, he's free to do that or anything else he likes as long as he's safe and not creating a disturbance in the village in the middle of the night.

We've also found the miracle of music. Bob's words mostly make no sense, but when he relaxes on the veranda and the boys put on compilation CDs of Nat King Cole, Frank Sinatra, Ella Fitzgerald, Frankie Lane and other crooners from his youth, his normally dull eyes well up with light and he sings along with them.

One day I'm sitting at Batan Waru waiting for the caregivers to bring Bob for our appointed lunch date. I've ordered our food ahead, hoping to waylay some of his anxiety about having to wait once we order. My cellphone rings.

"Bob doesn't want to go. He says he has work to do," Asa tells me. My shoulders tense. "When I told him you'd be there he said, 'Fine, you go. I have too much work.' He seems anxious."

I take a deep breath. "Listen Wayan, put on Bob's music and I'll get the food to-go. We can eat there."

When I walk through the cottage gate I hear Sinatra's voice coming from inside the house. Daisy greets me, jumping up and down and practically knocking the food boxes out of my hands. I set them on the table on the veranda and peek in the doorway. There's Bob, stark naked, stretched out on the couch, singing along with Frank. He can't carry on a conversation any longer, but he still knows the words to these songs.

"Is that any way to greet a lady?" I joke as I bend down to kiss him. He pats the cushion for me to sit next to him and takes my hand. After a few more songs, I say, "Why don't you put some clothes on and I'll get lunch on the table."

Bob appears a few minutes later, trying to cinch his belt. He has nothing else on. I turn away so he won't see me giggling. Asa gets him into a pair of shorts before he digs into his favorite chicken curry.

Nano, Ketut, Asa, and Krok are more than caregivers; they've become family to Bob. They tell me he's happier in the cottage than when he was in our home. They've learned not to say, 'No,' to Bob, but only redirect when necessary. I'm supremely grateful for the job they do - they're lifesavers for both of us.

***

More Alz Angels come into our life in 2012 in the form of a French couple on honeymoon in Bali. Both are psychologists who work with people with Alzheimer's and their caregivers. They teach us how important lighting is and how shadows create anxiety for people with dementia because they can't distinguish the subtle differences within them. They tell us that if you paint a black line on the floor, an Alzheimer's patient will step over it because they perceive it as a hole.

Alan generously spends six hours one day putting in new lights for Bob. Now all his rooms have bright light, eliminating most shadows, and his caregivers make sure the lamps are turned on well before the afternoon sun begins to wane. The garden is now lit all night, so when Bob gets up for a wee hour pee and peeks through the blinds, outside looks familiar instead of being a dark, scary space that gives him no clues to where he is. His caregivers report he's less anxious, sleeps longer in the night, and is less incontinent, and they're sure it's due to this simple lighting solution.

We also learn the value of color from the French couple, who tell us that if you want the person to go through a door, paint it a different color than the wall. If, on the other hand, you don't want them to open a door, paint it the same color as the wall. We immediately paint each room a different color so Bob can tell where he is. His bedroom becomes lilac, the TV room is light blue-grey, the bathroom yellow and the kitchen and veranda, where he spends most of the day, his favorite color – baby blue. We hang blue curtains over the under-the-counter shelves so he won't be tempted to snack on the dog treats or 'organize' items we need to find.

Often, Alzheimer's patients don't eat enough. We learn that putting food on a contrasting colored plate, such as putting mashed potatoes on a red plate, encourages them to eat more., Fortunately, Bob still has a hearty appetite. Our French friends also explain that by noticing what Bob already likes to do, we can create activities that will let him feel useful and enhance his sense of dignity. Bob spends a lot of time 'organizing' things, including the dishes, so I buy him various brightly-colored plastic dishes and bowls to organize to his heart's content.

Bob loves tools and always had a plethora of them. Alan and I spend a playful afternoon shopping for and filling a canvas tote with the word 'Tools' printed on it. We fill it with wrenches, nuts and bolts, a tape measure, and other cheap, safe tools he can do no damage with either to himself or others. Bob spends hours with this bag, taking everything out and scrutinizing it and finally putting it all back in. He does this day in and day out.

'The Alzheimer's Reading Room', my favorite blog, suggests stuffed animals as another way to give the person something to do and alleviate anxiety through tactile sensations. I'm apprehensive about this because I don't want Bob to feel he's being treated like a child, but finally decide to give it a try. I choose a soft, fuzzy shorebird, a tern about twelve inches long, for his stuffed animal. He bonds with it immediately and takes it to bed that night. Soon, he's carrying it around, petting it, and sometimes throwing it at the caregivers. When I tell Victoria this story she says, as she's been saying for years, "I hope you're writing this all down."

For months I've been thinking about creating a blog on my experiences as an Alzheimer's caregiver. I've kept putting it off, wondering, *What do I have to offer when there are other sites, such as The Alzheimer's Reading Room*? Then one day while I'm working on my professional site I notice a button marked

'New Blog'. I click to check it out, that click leads to other clicks, and before I know it, I've started 'Alz World – stories of caregiving written with the hope to inspire other caregivers of people with dementia as their stories have inspired me.'

***

Late that summer I go to the States for Bob's grandson's wedding and to empty out our storage trailer while the weather's warm, a job too difficult in the cold of winter. It's time to face what I've been dreading - the remnants of storage from 1987, when we first went to Asia, and the final deconstruction of our old life.

I've known for years that Bob would never use the myriad of tools stored there: some Bob's, some from both of our fathers. I knew he'd never wear the winter clothes or admire my artwork that used to mystify him. "How do you come up with these images?" Mr. Plain Vanilla would query with each new painting.

Buried in my art drawers, I find a series of colored pencil drawings. Clearly, they're mine, but strangely, I have no recollection of creating them. Nestled among those pages is a card from Bob, written in Malaysia in the early 90's. It reads:

"I love you and our life together.

I'll follow you to islands and places till I drop in my tracks.

When I do drop, please don't stop traveling your path.

I'm enjoying finding my path, growth, awakening with you.

Love, Bob"

This card feels like a blessing urging me to move on, to dissolve our old life knowing the memories of the love we shared will always remain. That love inspires me to do my best to make his life with Alzheimer's as comfortable as possible, but also to sashay down my own path, opening to new possibilities with this treasured benediction.

***

2013 brings many changes. Burned out with caregiving, Nano moves on to other work. A new man, Gusti, takes the job. He'd worked with Ketut caring for a man in a wheelchair for eight years and taken care of an elderly man with mild dementia who was unable to care for himself, and had recently passed away.

Gusti is hands on with Bob, and his sense of humor frequently gets Bob laughing. One day Bob says to me, "That's a good man!" It touches me that he still recognizes that quality and is clearly fond of his newest caregiver. Gusti seems born for this work.

On April 26, 2013, Bob turns eighty-one. He still looks more than a decade younger. We meet at Batan Waru to celebrate over lunch. The staff greets Bob with handshakes and pats on the back as he stumbles in – he's been having difficulties with balance in the last year. At the end of the meal they come out of the kitchen singing and bearing a small cake with a flaming candle. Bob hasn't forgotten what to do, and blows it out to applause. He's beaming.

It's been thirteen years since I almost died of a strangulated intestine and we first suspected something was seriously wrong with him. Since then, the Bob I married has shattered and splintered. Yet I know his essence is still there even though well-meaning friends advise me that no one is home anymore.

A week after his birthday I go for a visit. Sadly, his communication skills have declined to the point where I frequently have no idea what he's trying to convey. I smile and nod, patting his arm or stroking his shoulder to give him reassurance. Gripped by dense sadness over what this disease has taken from him, I have to muster all my courage not to weep in his presence.

This particular day he seems worried about our 'stuff' and about strangers who might come in and take things from us. Sitting together, we have tea, cookies and a banana and I nonchalantly set a plastic container with separate compartments on the table. I'd put objects like clothespins, tiny plastic dishes and a ball inside. I know his curiosity will get the better of him and he'll investigate it. What I haven't anticipated is that he'll try to put his peeled banana in it.

As I'm about to leave, I ask Ketut, "Now, what was it that Bob needs?"

In a strong voice, Bob yells, "SEX!" It's the old Bob spirit coming to the fore, a reminder that he's still in there. His brain is abandoning him, his body is failing, his life has pared down to a small cottage with a dog, four caregivers and a wife. But inside, behind the thick curtain of Alzheimer's, Bob's essence still lives.

A month later he comes down with pneumonia. His oldest daughter, Michele, who's a paramedic, comes from Hawaii because we think this might be the end. After six days in hospital, his chest x-ray shows his lungs are much worse than when he was admitted. Michele and I decide to bring him home. But miraculously he improves, falls back, then improves some more until he's starting to walk again and can even shower unassisted.

This rollercoaster leaves me with sleepless nights, acid stomachaches, and grief, making it difficult to think and function during the day. It brings up a lot of angst, life and death questions, and uncomfortable dark corners in my psyche. Once he's home and getting better, the panic subsides and I realize I hadn't been ready to let him go.

My husband's been an anchor to my life from the time we fell in love on Filicudi. We dove into the depths of our psyches with Helen and Lisa, journeyed through Southeast Asia and India, then birthed and built our mammoth tusk carving business together in Bali. Being married to Bob and being a caregiver is part of my identity.

I'd been ill the day before Bob got pneumonia and the caregivers didn't want to bother me, so took him to the clinic on their own. The doctor called me, wanting to give him antibiotics, and that was the first I knew he was ill. I agreed to the medication. They also advised me to hospitalize him.

It was after he was admitted that I dug out Bob's Advanced Medical Directive, buried in our file cabinet. It had been years since I'd read this document, which he'd made nineteen years before. It stunned me to see his handwriting stating that if he had a terminal illness, was dependent on others, and unable to make decisions for himself, he didn't want to be given antibiotics or hydration, and no resuscitation if he was in critical condition.

He'd seen the devastation Alzheimer's wrought on his mother and two of her sisters. He only wanted to be kept comfortable, and out of pain if possible and allowed to die.

I grapple with my earlier decision to allow hydration and antibiotics. I'm a wreck, not sleeping well and panicked at the thought I might lose Bob. I realize I have work to do on myself because I can't keep him alive selfishly. Yet watching my soulmate gasping for breath horrified me. I knew the medication would take that away. I considered stopping it while he was in hospital, but I couldn't bring myself to do that. Michele agreed. Hydration and antibiotics felt like comfort care.

Sadly, over the next five months Bob has two bouts of dehydration that leave him permanently unable to walk, completely incontinent, and unable to feed himself. People with Alzheimer's don't know when they're thirsty, and therefore, often don't drink enough. I know this is the start of the end. I'm so sure of this that I contact a cremation company and put into place what will be needed if he doesn't make it until I return from my annual shows in the States.

Margie, Alan and Made, my office manager, are with me when Agus, the very gentle and sweet funeral director, comes to the house with forms and procedures for a foreigner dying in Bali. He'll take care of everything - dealing with the US Consulate, arranging the documentation, picking up the body, washing and dressing Bob and contacting family and friends if need be. He'll hold the ashes until I return and then organize a boat to scatter them a few hundred yards out to sea. All for $2000.

I'm listening and filling out forms with a matter of fact focus. Then, suddenly, the tears come. Margie puts her arm around me and Alan takes my hand. Later, I pick out the clothes I want Bob to be cremated in and put them in the closet, well marked. I choose a tan silk shirt we'd had made for him in Bombay as a symbol of our time with Ramesh. There's a pair of silk Thai fisherman pants because our whole life in Asia was born in Bangkok's Chatuchak Market, where the pants came from, and because Bob loved the sea. Onto the hanger I put his favorite bear head necklace, made from fossil walrus tusk strung on a cord with ancient Middle Eastern glass beads. Onto the necklace I slip the silver and amethyst engagement ring that he bought for me on a trip to England in 1985. I hold his clothes to my nose, and even though they've been in the closet for three years, I can smell his smell. I weep.

On the January day I leave for the States, I go to see him and find him napping on his bed. I climb up next to him, stretch out alongside with my hand on his chest over his heart and adjust my breathing to match his. He stirs a bit but never fully wakes up while I whisper how much I love him, fighting back tears. It feels like the final good-bye.

***

In my absence I've offered my house to my grandniece, Julie, who works as a nurse in the States but will be in Ubud for several weeks while I'm gone. She arrives in mid-February, makes time to visit Bob, and brings him a root beer float – one of his favorite treats. Then she emails me a photo of Bob beaming as she spoons the cold delight into his mouth.

In early March after my shows are finished, I stay with my sister in northern California while I gather supplies to take back to Bali. We're watching a movie one evening when Made calls. Bob is in the clinic with pneumonia again. The doctor wants to send him to the hospital. I quickly confer with his daughters and we're all in agreement: this time no hospital and no antibiotics.

I feel so far away and so conflicted about whether or not I should go back to Bali immediately or continue doing what I need to do and go as scheduled. Bob could hang on again and get better, and I have so many loose ends that need tying up before I leave. I receive an email from Heather, one of the Goddesses, who's gone to see Bob. Heather has nursing experience and she writes that she's done some Buddhist prayers for him, but in her opinion he's not ready to go. This helps me decide to stay and finish up.

I email Julie the latest Bob news. She's gone to a nearby island for some beach fun with friends. As soon as she gets the email, she calls me and says, "I'm preparing to return to Ubud on the next boat." I feel a mix of relief and concern that I'm ruining her vacation. "Susan, I'm an ICU nurse – this is what I do! I'm good at being with people at the end of life. It's sort of a calling."

I start to cry, so grateful that this angel – yes, another angel in our lives - is willing to drop everything and care for Bob. If I can't be there, at least Julie can, and we're blood-related; this feels important to me.

Julie spends her first night back in Ubud sitting with Bob, trying to keep him comfortable and helping Gusti turn him so he won't get bedsores. In the next week she's frequently at his bedside. I get daily emails keeping me up to date. Miraculously, he's getting better. Sometimes it feels like he'll outlive us all.

But the day I arrive in Bali, Bob stops eating. I go to him. He's mostly unconscious but occasionally groans or flutters his eyes. At one point he looks right at me and I feel there's recognition. I need to believe there's recognition – that I'm not too late. I feel strongly he's waited for me.

I pull my chair up as close to him as I can get and spend the day stroking his forehead, his arm, his chest, and holding his hand. I tell him stories of our life together, of our great love, what a perfect husband he's been and how we'll always be connected. He burbles with every difficult breath. A doctor and nurse come from the clinic and hook him up to an IV so we can add painkillers as needed to keep him as comfortable as possible. This eases his breathing and my distress.

Julie stops by to see how we're doing. I feel her compassion and caring in the way she talks to Bob and the warm hugs she's so generous with. I try to contact Bob's daughters, and though I can't reach Dawn, Skype brings Michele into the room. When she talks to her dad, he stirs. I'm convinced he knows who she is. She tells him what a great dad he's been and how much she loves him. She tells him that it's OK to go. We'll be fine.

This time there's no turning back, no miraculous healing as happened the previous year. The end is near.

***

The next day Margie stops in to say goodbye. Bob is slipping further and further away. Gusti tells me that the man he cared for before Bob lasted like this for a week; I relax a bit, sure that Bob is not yet ready to leave. But at five the next morning he stops breathing.

Julie and I rush over, picking up Margie along the way. The doctor is already there making the legal pronouncement. All the caregivers gather and the seven of us bathe Bob, dressing him in the clothes I'd picked out in January. We cover him with his favorite antique Javanese batik sarong, soft from decades of hand washing. He'd worn this to countless temples and ceremonies in Bali; now it would accompany him to the ultimate ceremony.

The cottage fills with people. My landlords, Bob's landlord, our neighbours Jean and William, our staff, and other friends come to say good-bye. Asa and Ketut make coffee for everyone and serve Balinese pastries that Krok has rushed out to buy. Daisy, the dashhound, looks lost. Margie holds me as I weep.

My landlord puts an offering of coffee, pastry, sandalwood incense, rice and flower petals next to Bob to accompany him on his journey. I pick flowers from the garden and put them behind his ears and in his hands. Margie picks a bouquet of flowers and colorful leaves and places them in a cut-off plastic water bottle. We all make do with what's on hand, everyone wanting to do something for this man who touched us all. I sense Bob is still with us, watching his body cool and the hive of subdued activity around it.

Agus, the cremation director, shows up with an ambulance and a team of four sturdy men. When I'm ready, they respectfully lift Bob onto the stretcher and take him away. The house feels so empty.

That afternoon I make an altar using photos of Bob, a crystal from our wedding, a favorite bracelet of his, an oversized book of Buddhist paintings and a wooden statue of Kuan Yin that Victoria gave him for a long ago birthday. Kuan Yin is the Asian Goddess of Compassion. I add a picture of Ramesh and then very carefully set a lit candle in a glass holder in front of this collection. I put it close, but away from the photos, remembering how we lost everything to a candle so many years ago.

In the middle of the night I wake up tossing and turning. I start thinking about the candle and the possibility that the house and my life could go up in sparks, and Julie in the bedroom along with it. I lie there trying to calm my mind, telling myself that the candle would have burned down to its bottom hours ago.

But when I get up in the morning, shivers run through me when I see one of my favorite photos of Bob has come unfastened and fallen over the candleholder. The flame burned about a fifth of the photo away, but stopped when it came into contact with the edge of the glass holder. I shudder as I realize how close we came to disaster. I feel Bob is protecting us, and that he somehow had a hand in this.

The caregivers take turns sleeping in pairs at the mortuary for the next three nights because they don't want to leave Bob alone. I'm tearfully grateful for this. But I have to pull myself together and notify everyone who might want to come to the cremation. It's a big job for a muddled mind.

On the day of the cremation, three carloads of friends arrive to accompany Bob to the crematorium, an hour's drive through dense city traffic. We're met by friends already gathered there. Bob's photo is placed on top of the casket with a rope of large marigold flowers draped around it. More people filter in, about half Balinese and half Western, till there are sixty of us. I'm touched that so many Balinese have come.

Agus removes the casket's lid and everyone who wants to, sprinkles handfuls of flower petals over the length of Bob's body. He's covered in rose, bougainvillea, frangipani, and hydrangea petals before the top is replaced. Then the casket is slid into the furnace.

Agus asks if I want to push the button to start the burners. I hesitate, my mind in a surreal fog, but something - it doesn't feel exactly like me - decides this experience should not be missed and I wave others up to share in this send-off. As many hands as can be are on my hand, arm and shoulders, while others touch the shoulders of those in front until everyone is daisy-chained through the open air hall. I push the button. The burners ignite.

***

Michele and her daughter Niki arrive from Hawaii a week later, in time for Bob's memorial and the scattering of his ashes out at sea. Dawn and her family can't make it. Sixty of us meet at a seaside cafe to celebrate Bob with stories, sweets, lemon drop martinis, tears and laughter. His dancing shoes are on the altar we've set up for him with a backdrop filled with photos from his life. There are flowers everywhere. Leis of frangipani and marigold strung together by Niki and our staff are set on all the tables, there's a beautiful arrangement of red and pink torch ginger and red anthuriums amid hen and chick succulents from the Goddesses on the altar table. White bougainvillea bedecks the drinks table.

Linda officiates the gathering, now in a semi-circle of chairs. The few words I try to speak get caught in my throat. People stand up to tell stories about Bob or read letters sent by those who can't be present like the one from friends we'd made on that first trip to Asia, Jette and Phillip:

'Jette and I have a photograph of Bob and Susan standing on the beach on Tioman Island, looking out to sea, waiting for their boat to take them to their next destination back in '87. Bob, back then, was in his mid-fifties, and standing on that beach, he cut a stunning figure. For us ordinary men, Bob was your usual nightmare; he had the sculptured looks of a Greek god, but with a Californian attitude, a soft baritone voice, beautiful hands and a wonderful sense of humor. His delivery of one-liners followed by that broad, manly smile simply disarmed everyone. But for me personally, I will remember Bob for 3 things. Firstly, his tenderness and generosity that led to our friendship with Bob and Susan when Bob generously gave a stranger, Jette, a neck and shoulder massage and relieved her of the pain she was going through and then showed me how to do it. Secondly, sitting alone with him on the terrace of their house in Ubud under a mosquito net watching fireflies dance over the paddy fields, not saying a word. That evening Bob taught me the art of doing absolutely nothing and simply enjoying it. Finally, and most importantly, the love that Bob and Susan showered upon one another has been a constant inspiration to Jette and myself the past 28 years. We will miss him dearly. Jette and Phillip'

After the stories, we toast Bob with lemon drop martinis and file over to the beach where there's some confusion as a boat unloads its cargo of cattle into the surf and men pull them to shore. Then two traditional *prahu* come to take fourteen of us out into the calm sea. We mirror the bovine confusion, with friends unsure who should go with the family and staff. I vaguely know this is going on, but I've made it clear I can't make decisions today – someone else will have to do it. In the end everyone who really wants to go wades through the waves and climbs into one of the boats.

The Balinese believe that the soul can't reincarnate until this last part of the cremation ceremony is complete – returning the last vestiges of a person to the sea. No ashes are allowed to be kept. If the family can't get to the shore, they sprinkle the ashes in a river that empties into the ocean. Bob had always wanted the sea to take his ashes wherever he died.

Ketut has prepared a Balinese farewell offering in a square basket; he adds sticks of burning sandalwood incense to the rice, flowers, fruit, cloth and palm leaf container inside, then recites prayers over it in a focused manner. Gently, he sets the basket down to float in the sea, accompanying Bob on his journey 'home'.

Becol, our production manager, Michele, Niki, and I, sprinkle flower petals on the water. Then we take handfuls of ashes and pure white bits of bone and cast them to the breeze. It's a fitting parting for such a gallant man. I feel gratitude, blessing, and joy for this beautiful day dedicated to my soul mate, for the life we shared, and for the love showered on us by our friends and family.

***

Two days after the memorial, a newly-hatched chick wanders into our yard. She's a piece of tiny black fluff cheeping around the garden and we worry a predator will get her. The staff ask around, but no one knows where she came from and no one has lost her. We look for a mother hen, but she's the only chicken in our vicinity.

The chick creeps nearer and nearer as she forages in the plants around the house until one evening she bolts into the kitchen and under the stove. When a visiting Balinese friend throws himself on the floor and reaches under the oven to pull her out, she bonds with us immediately. By the next day we can pick her up and handle her. She's not afraid of any of us.

Not being a bird person, I don't know what to feed her, so I try some of Bob's favorite homemade muesli. She loves it, and when she learns to fly, she flies up onto the counter and pecks only on the canister with this muesli even though there are other jars and bottles. We name her MillyBob, unsure whether she's a hen or a cock, but sensing she's female.

MillyBob follows me like a dog and perches on my shoulder while I'm at the computer or dining table. She also attaches herself to Alan. My staff are sure she's connected with Bob. The Balinese believe in reincarnation, and that they're born again and again into the same family line. While I'm not Hindu and I don't believe as they do, I have a sense that MillyBob, in some magical way, has been sent to us.

While she's small, the chick wants to be on our hands, arms, shoulders, and occasionally the tops of our heads, but her favorite spot becomes the top of the computer monitor, where she nestles down to preen while I work, downy feathers floating between us. I have to warn her not to peck at the cursor. She coos and chirps chicken songs in my ear when she's on the back of my chair at breakfast or lunch. Before the sun sets every evening, we put her in large basket with a perch, water, food and a straw nest where she's safe and content.

Milly feels like a gift that helps dispel the sadness, especially after Julie, Michele and Niki leave and Alan goes back to work in Malaysia. She makes us all laugh and becomes such a boon to the house that I don't mind cleaning up after her.

***

Sitting on my file cabinet is the photo of Bob that my staff had printed and framed for his cremation. It has smudges on it where the long-gone marigold garland has rubbed away the print. He's sitting cross-legged on a low sofa in a beach bar in Bombay on one our Ramesh trips, beaming broadly at me and the camera, so handsome and at home in his body. I often find myself talking to that photo, saying, "Good-night Bob!" or "Beautiful day, isn't it?" or "Thanks for Milly." He feels so much a part of me still. It's like he's everywhere, even in the air I breathe.

THE END

In Gratitude

So many people touched our lives and helped us through this challenging disease. I also want to thank everyone who had a say in this book and who inspired me to go on with it. These acknowledgments are not in any particular order – everyone was important on this journey. For anyone I've missed - my deepest apologies – it wasn't intentional.

To Hanna and Keith – the first Alz angels who taught Nano, Ketut and me that we didn't need to reinvent the wheel. Without their knowledge and caring we couldn't have pulled this off. Sadly Hanna passed away in December 2010.

To Dr. Susila – Bob's Balinese primary care physician who made house calls whenever asked and who sadly passed away from cancer in 2012.

To Michele and Dawn – Bob's daughters who stepped up to the plate and were there for us both.

To Ketut Sama, Gusti, Wayan Asa, Nano, and Ketut Krok, – caregivers extraordinaire, whose unending patience and quick thinking allowed us to give Bob the best life possible.

To Joan – my adoring and adorable sister who patiently listened to all my trials and tribulations with love and wisdom and continues to do so.

To Cat – whose quiet support and brilliant ideas saved me on several occasions

To Dorene, Victoria and Vicki – who encouraged me to keep going and keep writing.

To Mary – for years of Sunday brunches watching Bob descend into Alz World and being a steady support.

To Margie – whose enduring love and friendship buoyed me up when I was drowning.

To Kristi – my kind, patient, talented editor who inspired me to strip away the excess, reorganize the remainder, and add what was missing. She COULD see the forest for the trees.

To Jean and William – my neighbors and dear friends who watched this unfold from twenty feet away and were there for me whenever I needed them.

To the Ubud Goddesses - my martini group who kept me laughing when all I wanted to do is cry. Laughter is a great healer. Friendship a great support.

To Ramesh Balsekar - who gave me the spiritual foundation to endure this challenge and find peace in whatever happens.

To Alan - for bringing romance and love back into my life, helping with Bob, and keeping me sane

To Ganesha – for removing obstacles

Resources

American Alzheimer's Association

(http://www.alz.org)

The Alzheimer's Reading Room – my favorite resource for caregiving, with thousands of articles

(http://www.alzheimersreadingroom.com)

Research on letting Alzheimer's patients do what they want when they want (http://legacy.king5.com/story/news/health/2014/08/02/13009710/)

How music helps Alzheimer's patients

(http://www.npr.org/2012/04/18/150891711/for-elders-with-dementia-music-sparks-great-awakenings)

More stories about caring for Bob and lessons learned on my blog:

www.alzworld-susantereba.blogspot.com

About the Author

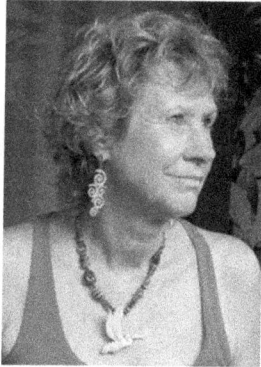

Susan Tereba is an American artist, jewelry designer and writer who came to live in Bali, Indonesia with her husband, Bob, in 1990. Ten years later he showed the first signs of Alzheimer's disease. For fourteen years Susan was Bob's primary caregiver, giving him the best life possible while keeping him with her in Bali.